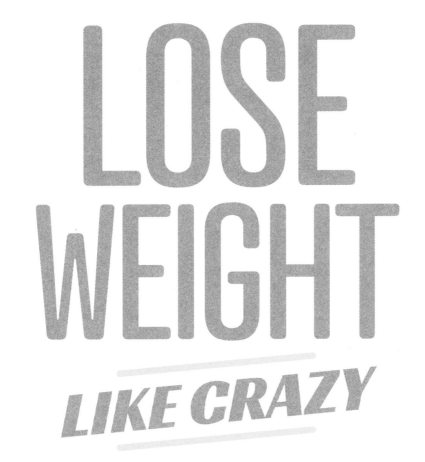

LOSE WEIGHT
LIKE CRAZY

LOSE WEIGHT

LIKE CRAZY

Even if You Have a Crazy Life!

AUTUMN CALABRESE

This book is intended as a general reference volume only, not as any form of medical treatment or advice. The information given here is designed to help you make informed decisions about your health and wellness. It is not provided or intended as any form of a medical diagnosis or plan, or a substitute for any treatment that may have been prescribed by your doctor.

If you have any unique medical issues or conditions, or otherwise suspect that you may have a medical issue or sensitivity, please first consult with a medical provider before starting this or any other nutrition program to discuss your specific needs.

Design by Galvanized Media
Library of Congress Cataloging-in-Publication Data
Name: Calabrese, Autumn, author.
Lose Weight Like Crazy Even If You Have a Crazy Life!
Life Lessons and a Breakthrough 30-Day Nutrition and Fitness Solution!
Autumn Calabrese
Los Angeles, CA

ISBN-13: 978-1-940358-51-2   **33614082927467**

Published by Beachbody LLC

www.beachbody.com

Recipe photography and creative direction by Jake Repko, CNW Agency; food styling and art direction by Hailee Repko, CNW Agency; food stylist: Angeline Woo, EL OJO Agency; stylist assistant: Brian Arnold.

Distributed to the book trade by Galvanized Media and Simon & Schuster

I dedicate this book to my family,
each and every crazy member. Without
all of you, I would not be the me I am today.
Thank you for the love & the lessons.
A special thank-you to my dad
who taught me to follow my dreams
no matter what anyone says.

CONTENTS

I LOST A CRAZY AMOUNT OF WEIGHT

Autumn Calabrese changed my life.

I am 35 years old and I would say 27 years of my life have been spent in a battle with my weight. You name the diet—I have probably tried it . . . more than once and failed at it. Nothing ever came easy, nothing ever made sense. I would try something new and got bored of it—which then led to gaining even more weight.

Growing up I was made to feel bad about myself because of my weight and eating habits. I would be forced into certain diets that never made me feel good. They left me feeling either sick, starving, or extremely bloated. There was never a consistent pattern in any of the "diets" I was on. It was either eat a pound of broccoli and fish, or you can eat greasy burgers and mayo but no bun. How was any of that sustainable or going to make me be able to lose weight the healthy way? It wasn't.

I feel like I've been on a diet for as long as I can remember. My mother created fears about weight and taught me, "You can never be too thin." I've battled with this idea my entire life, which has led to dietary changes and always seeking a quick fix. To me the word "diet" has always been a punishment and was never made a choice. It was never something I did for myself, but to appease the views of others.

All of the other diets I have been on have always been about losing weight and never taught me the value of nutrition and healthy eating. They were just a means to facilitate an outside appearance that would have been seen as acceptable by those closest to me.

In 2018 I became the unhealthiest I've ever been. I am a wife, and a mom of 2 amazing boys (Owen, 6, and Caden, 2). I would eat fast food 4 or 5 times a week and then throw out the bags to hide the evidence from my family. I had become lazy in making healthy meals that I would just throw together without thinking of nutrition. I had fallen back into so many bad habits that led to me feeling sad all day long. I hated the way I looked, how I felt, and, more importantly, the path I was heading down if I didn't change what I was doing.

November 2018 was when my life changed forever. It was when I asked for help and was introduced to Autumn and *The Ultimate*

Portion Fix. I needed to know what people were doing to get these amazing results. I needed to know all about it—NOW!

I jumped in. I watched all of the *Ultimate Portion Fix* videos, read all of the program materials, and used the workbooks and logbooks provided. There was no cutting out carbs or fruits like so many "diets" make you do. This made sense. There was no weighing my food or counting calories. I didn't have to give up foods that I love. I just had to pick healthier versions and proper portion sizes—something we all know but are never fully aware of how to do. I wish I would have known about this years ago—but what was important was that I had the tools I needed now.

The first few days I measured, I prepared meals ahead of time, and I used the tools Autumn had given me to set me up for success. Did I have doubts? Of course! I had doubts this was going to work for me—because nothing in the past had. But, I continued to measure, I continued to portion my meals and eat exactly how I was supposed to. My cravings for sugar slowly went away and it got easier. I was learning to cook healthy meals for my family! I realized this wasn't like anything I had ever done. I was able to eat all the food I normally would, but now I was using these containers as my guide and they taught me how to eat all over again.

Did I have a glass of wine? YES, but I would substitute a yellow container for it. Did I miss having sweets? No, because I was still able to make a delicious dessert from the long list of recipes on Autumn's cooking show *FIXATE*, all developed by her brother,

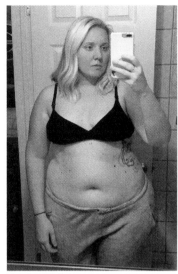
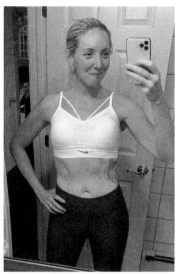

Day 1: 256 lbs.

Day 330*: 146 lbs.

"I lost 110 pounds and 18 inches off my waist!"

—**Jennifer H.**, 34, Independent Team
Beachbody Coach, Toms River, NJ

Chef Bobby Calabrese. Meal prepping had become so easy because all I had to do was measure everything in the containers.

I took this day by day, meal by meal. Month after month I would see the weight coming off, but more importantly, I felt the healthiest I ever have. Those containers travel with me if I leave the house, and they will never leave my pantry. I owe my health and so much of my happiness to Autumn and those containers, which is why I will never stop following this program. It has become so much more than that—this program has truly been life changing.

It has not only changed my life, it has changed my family's life. My older son will ask me if he is making a healthy choice or ask to be involved in cooking dinner. I am able to teach my sons what I know about nutrition and eating the best foods to properly fuel their bodies. I know what foods make me feel good and it's my job now to teach them the same thing. For so long I thought that eating healthy meant it tasted bland and boring—this isn't the case. *Portion Fix* is so much more than a container system—it is a life-changing program. It has given me so many resources that are continuously changing to create new and delicious meals for my family.

In one year I lost 110 pounds following Autumn's *Portion Fix* program and pushing play on her workouts. I used the tools that were given to me and followed them. There were no shortcuts, there was no easy way out. I knew I needed to change my old habits to see new results—long-lasting results. So, that's exactly what I did! I filled my containers and I listened to Autumn. When it got hard, I would remember her talking about our "why"s. Why was I doing this? To lose weight and be healthy. Why did I NEED to do this? Because I didn't want to die young. I wanted to grow old with my husband and watch my boys grow up. Those answers are ALWAYS in the back of my head.

My boys watch me push play to Autumn's workout programs every day and see me have fun doing it! I am able to make them delicious, healthy meals, and what is even more amazing is that they are aware of making healthy choices. A year ago, they were watching me sit around on a couch all day feeling sad and eating junk food. Today, they have the best version of me and it's all because of those 6 amazing containers.

—Jennifer Hennessey

When I started writing a book on how to lose weight like crazy even if you have a crazy life, I never could have imagined that just months before its launch we would be in the midst of the COVID-19 global pandemic. It's by far the craziest thing I've ever experienced in my life. This brings new meaning to the title of this book. When the virus started in Wuhan, China, it felt like a world away, something that we would hear about but wouldn't actually affect us here in the United States. First came the advice to wash our hands, and cough or sneeze into our elbow. Then came "social distancing," next we were asked to work from home if at all possible. Before we knew it, schools were closing, businesses were shutting down, and then the shelter-in-place orders swept the country. As I said, this is a global pandemic; the world is trying to adjust to a new "normal" while we work to get a handle on this crazy situation. There is fear and anxiety around the unknown, frustration from being cooped up indoors. People have lost their jobs, lost their loved ones, lost their positive outlook on life. We are being forced to figure out how to work from home, how to be teachers to our kids while working from home, how to take care of our elders without endangering them. The principles I'm teaching in this book are more important than ever. Losing weight like crazy amidst a crazy life isn't about 6-pack abs or bulging biceps; those things are fun but it's truly about taking back control of your health. I don't know how long this crisis will go on, I don't know what life will look like in the coming months and years, but here is what I do know:

1) Now, more than ever, it's imperative to take care of our health, to exercise regularly and fuel our bodies properly. Not just for our physical well-being, but for our emotional and mental well-being, as well.

2) This too shall pass.

We have the opportunity to come out stronger on the other side of this, just like with all crazy hard situations, but we have to take control of the things that we can right now. I'm being asked to write articles on what or how people can eat to be healthier, to create workouts that people can do at home that can be posted and shared. Life will always throw us curveballs, hopefully they won't be asteroid-sized ones like this very often but we always have 2 ways of handling the hard. We can lean into it, embrace it, and allow ourselves to grow and become better or we can buckle under it, succumb to it, and allow it to defeat us. I don't know about you but no matter how many times I get knocked down, I get up and come back swinging. I'm not going down without a fight. If you're here to fight for your health and your happiness, then I'm here to help.

—Autumn

LET'S GET CRAZY HEALTHY

What's up, Team AC.

Yes, you are now officially part of my team, and on my team, no one is left behind. Thanks for picking up my book. Just by taking this small step, you're saying you are ready to make big changes, to let go of the excuses and embrace the solution to living a CRAZY healthy, amazing life WITHOUT having to follow a CRAZY diet.

Let me tell you why I wrote this book for you:

- To teach you that healthy eating isn't actually all that hard.

- To show you how to eat what you love and lose weight like crazy (or just be crazy healthy).

- To prove that even with the craziest life, you CAN do it.

Ever since I was a kid, my life has been nothing short of crazy. Don't believe me? Read on. But, despite all the crazy, I've ended up here: a fitness and nutrition expert, certified health and wellness coach, and one of the best-selling Beachbody Super Trainers in the company's history. When I launched my first program, *21 Day Fix*, it sold on its first day what Beachbody had projected to sell in its first week. In its first week, it outsold projections for the first month. And after its first month, we sold out and were on back order for 3 months! That was my first fitness and nutrition program. CRAZY! Since then, I've had a string of hits that you might know of: *21 Day Fix Extreme, The Master's Hammer & Chisel* resistance training system, *Country Heat*, a low-impact, country music–based dance workout, *80 Day Obsession, Ultimate Portion Fix*, and my cookbooks and cooking show *FIXATE*.

I should also let you know that I'm a single mom, and to live this amazing life takes a lot of work. To put out 8 fitness programs, 2 cookbooks, an ongoing cooking show, and a continually updated nutrition program in the last 7 years, all while taking care of my son and maintaining my own health, that ain't easy, but it also ain't impossible. It just takes a plan. A plan that I'm going to share with you. This is a beautiful, awesome, messy, blessed life that I am living, but make no mistake, it is still crazy!

I tell you all this not to brag about my accomplishments, but to shed light on your amazing potential in your own crazy, busy life. I'm also sharing the details of my present life to put my past in perspective, so you can see where I am NOW as you're about to learn where I came from, because that, too, is a crazy story.

You can ask me to do something or show me how to do something, but don't ever TELL me what to do. I don't like being TOLD what to do. I'm the youngest of 3 kids. My brother Bobby, sister Calie, and I were raised by our single dad in Collinwood, a little Italian neighborhood on the east side of Cleveland. Everyone knew Bobby Cal and everyone knew his kids because my dad owned the local pizza place, and in a little Italian neighborhood that kind of makes you a local celebrity.

My dad was an entrepreneur, and his pizza shop, Bobby Cal's, was not his first restaurant. He'd owned another just before I was born, in a small town called Barberton, but lost it when the local auto plant shut down and the town went into recession. My dad was a fighter, though, and he had mouths to feed, so for the next 2 years he ran a catering company out of my grandma's basement kitchen. This was the '80s in Cleveland, Ohio. Clearly that wouldn't fly now, but my dad made it work until he'd saved enough to reopen his restaurant once again. Watching him work long hours, watching him hustle, watching him build his dream is what ultimately taught me that I could do the same. My dad always said, "Do something you love, and you'll never work a day in your life."

Great advice, but here's the thing, my dad isn't just "a dad." He's an "Italian dad." His way is the only way.

So, while he taught us to dream big, he kept a short leash on my siblings and me. My brother, Bobby, worked in our restaurant at a very young age, 9, maybe 10 years old. (That's funny looking back at it now. My son is 10 and barely knows how to turn the stove on!) Bobby would go to the restaurant, and my sister Calie and I were left to take care of the house on the weekends. At 7 years old I didn't like being told I had to stay home and clean the house and do the laundry with my big sister. I wanted to play. During the week we all had responsibilities in the restaurant before school and after. I would make the antipasto salads for the to-go cooler, put the slices of cheesecake in their containers, make pizza boxes or restock the chips and soda. This was not for allowance, people. This is just what I was TOLD to do before and after school. I learned a work ethic at a very young age, but I also learned to eat pizza, pasta, cheesecake, and soda almost every day!

In grade school, I was never a straight-A student. I didn't particularly enjoy school, probably because I went to a Catholic school, and if anyone is known for TELLING you what to do it's the nuns at a Catholic grade school. I would daydream about being an actress, a dancer, or a model. I would play Madonna, Paula Abdul, and Janet Jackson and dance around the house nonstop. It drove everyone crazy. My dad would always say, "You're so peaceful when you sleep." I didn't know what that meant until I had my son, who is just as energetic as I was. Oh my gosh, where does that energy come from, and how do we get it back?

Anyway, I wanted to dance, I wanted to do everything, go everywhere, see everything. But we pretty much stayed in our little neighborhood bubble. I would go to school, do my homework, do my chores. When we'd go out to play it was always, "Only down to Stevenson Street and no farther than Mandalay! Be back at the house by sundown." OK, I was a kid and, yes, kids are basically told what to do, but I never liked it.

There were a lot of rules, a lot of things I wasn't allowed to do. Playdates rarely happened, a sleepover was next to impossible to schedule. I don't really remember going to friends' birthday parties. Like I said, Italian dad.

My dad made all 3 of us pick a musical instrument to play, and he signed us up for music lessons at the Cleveland Institute of Music. I didn't really pick; my dad picked the violin for me. I was 6 and my hands were too small to play a real violin, so my teacher started me with a crackerjack box that had a ruler taped to it so I could learn the hand positions. Bobby played the saxophone and clarinet, and Calie played the piano. We HAD to practice every day for an hour. When we were done with our chores, my dad would send us upstairs to practice. If he didn't hear us playing, he would yell up, "I don't hear you. That's 5 more minutes!" Looking back, I wish I appreciated it more but, again, I HATED being TOLD what to do.

That idea of hating being TOLD or talked at has stuck with me, and it's actually one of the main reasons I wanted to start my own business, as well as why I train people the way I do. I wanted to be my own boss, so no one could tell me what to do. I would be in control of my schedule, my time, the amount of money I made, and ultimately my life.

Let's jump ahead to college. I went to a small performing arts college in St. Louis, Missouri. In all honesty it's the only performing arts college I got into. I wanted to dance, but I started training much later than most girls. I never learned to dance ballet on pointe shoes, which are required for most college auditions. I was excited just to get into college with a major in dance. As a young dancer in Ohio, I had AMAZING dance teachers, teachers who built me up, gave me constructive criticism, taught the importance of taking care of our bodies, and, most importantly, made sure dance was always fun, even when we were competing.

So, there I was in my freshman year of college, excited to be at school DANCING. I LOVED jazz. Turn the music up and let me move. Ya, the head of my dance department didn't see it that way. Everyone was supposed to be a ballerina first. He always taught jazz class to techno music, which I hate, and choreography class . . . well they took us outside, said pick an object you see out here and create a dance about it. WTF? I don't dance because I see a tree, I dance because I hear a song, the beat, the rhythm, the lyrics that make me want to move. But here I was again being TOLD what was supposed to make me dance.

I could go on and on about bosses at jobs not asking, not showing but just telling. All of it creates a very deep, visceral, angry reaction in me. Hey, I'm human, and I'm being honest.

My Teaching Philosophy

So, what does all of this have to do with nutrition? Well I could TELL you to eat vegetables, drink water, don't eat crap, get enough sleep, take care of yourself. But let's be honest, would I be TELLING you something you don't already know? Yeah, probably not. It's human nature not to want to be talked down to, or to just be told do it this way because I said so. It's human nature to be curious, to want to understand why. This idea of why is going to come up a lot for us in different ways in this book. But understanding WHY we need to eat a certain way, understanding HOW that way of eating will benefit us, that is a plan you are much more likely to stick with. So, I'm not just going to tell you what to do. I'm going to let you into my life. I'm going to explain HOW I came up with the *Ultimate Portion Fix* method, WHY it works, and HOW it can work for you! I hope you are as excited as I am to go on this journey. It's going to be a hell of a ride. Something to keep in mind, this ride never ends. It's a way of eating, a way of fueling your body that can last a lifetime. This ride has ups and downs; it's fun and scary but ultimately, if you stick with it, it will lead to CRAZY AWESOME results.

Autumn Calabrese

As I take you on this ride, I'm going to give you "bite-size" challenges that you can do each day. That's because it's easier to conquer a bunch of small goals that culminate in accomplishing the big goal. Those little victories are important, don't sleep on them. Or do, if the challenge is getting more sleep that week! But just know they are there to empower you, to show you that you can do hard things, and that healthy nutrition isn't that hard after all.

CRAZY EASY, CRAZY POWERFUL **TIP #1**

Knowledge Is Power

It's important to know where you are in order to know where you're going. Write down everything you ate and drank today, every single thing, and write what time you had them. Write down how you felt physically and mentally/emotionally after each meal. Take a look at what you wrote at the end of the day. Where do you feel you have room for improvement? What do you think you are doing well? I'm going to teach you everything you need to know to follow my *Portion Fix* plan, but it's important for you to know where you're starting.

THE HONEST TRUTH ABOUT LOSING WEIGHT LIKE CRAZY

Over the past 5 years, I've simplified eating for hundreds of thousands of people with my breakthrough, color-coded container system and helped them become leaner, healthier, and happier versions of themselves. And now I'm going to do the same for you by teaching you my honest approach to good nutrition.

Yeah, I said honest because most weight-loss programs aren't so honest. If you've tried others, like I have, you know what I mean. They make a lot of bold promises for super-quick results that don't quite pan out, or they fizzle out after the initial weight loss. I'm going to give it to you straight because I respect you and I'm not here to waste your time.

If you came looking for a diet, sorry to disappoint. My program can get you crazy results crazy fast, but it's not a diet. It's a lifestyle designed to be able to follow forever, no matter the occasion or how crazy life gets. Again, It's NOT a DIET! Frankly, I can't stand the friggin' word. Most diets are all about saying no, no, no, no, no, and I'm not a fan of that word when it comes to my food. If you're going to tell me I shouldn't eat something, then you better have a damn good explanation as to why, 'cause I loooove food. Good

news, if I mention something that you shouldn't eat, I'll have
a damn good reason why.

Before I tell you what you should remove from your diet, let me
start with what you should add, H2O!

Drink More Water

Hydration is very important to your health. Your body is up to
60% water. If it's not properly hydrated, it can't function at optimum
levels. Let's start getting you hydrated. You should be drinking
half of your body weight in ounces of water every day.

That means if you weigh 200 pounds you should be drinking
a minimum of 100 ounces of water a day. Track your water intake
for a day to see how close you are to being properly hydrated.
If you're hitting your water intake each and every day, great, keep
up the good work. If you're nowhere near it, it's time to start
upping the H_2O. Get yourself a few glass or stainless steel water
bottles. I have a few 16-ounce travel stainless steel cups and
a few 32-ounce travel stainless steel cups. I NEVER leave home
without one, and at home, I always have a big glass of water
nearby. I also use metal straws. I find I drink more water when
I'm using a straw, but that might just be me. Start tracking how
many of your bottles or cups you drink a day. You can start slow—if
you haven't been drinking much water at all, you don't have to
jump right to 100 ounces—but you do want to get a little more in
each day until you are drinking half your body weight in ounces
of water a day.

Don't like water? Be aware that tap water can have a bad
taste, depending on where you live, so you might want to invest
in a water purifier that attaches to your kitchen sink or a water
purifier that you can refill and keep in your fridge. You can also try

adding fruit or vegetables like cucumbers and/or herbs to your water to flavor it up.

Try these infused waters: strawberry and blueberry, watermelon and basil, cucumber and mint.

Does all liquid count toward hydration? For our purposes the answer is no. Caffeinated beverages, like coffee and tea, do not count toward your water intake; neither does soda. Plain, filtered water, infused water, and unsweetened herbal tea count toward your water intake.

Back to the words "diet" and "no," and why I'm not a fan of either. The second someone tells me, "No, you can't eat pizza. No, you can't have chocolate," well, that's all I can think about: pizza and chocolate. I'll bet you're the same way. And here's what's even worse: the first time you fall off the diet wagon and eat that "taboo" food, you feel miserable, like a failure. Have you been there? I have. That's no way to live. It'll drive you crazy, but you certainly won't lose weight like CRAZY!

Diets of deprivation suck. And they don't work. They put you down the moment you stumble over some unrealistic requirement. Look, nobody likes to be told what to do and what they can't eat. Maybe that's why we have thousands of diets available to us, and yet, never before have we witnessed such an epidemic of diabetes and obesity. There are tons of diet books out there telling us: don't eat sugar, don't eat gluten, don't eat bread, don't eat meat, eat more meat, eat more fat, eat more protein, eat more nuts. I'm going nuts! Do this detox. Try this cleanse. Don't eat until Wednesday. WTF?

The failure of all these sure-fire weight-loss solutions is that they either miss the big picture or they don't want to tell you the truth. I'm going to level with you: We eat way too much food! That's the truth. We OVEREAT because we don't know how to gauge a realistic portion of food. We have food—mostly processed food—shoved in our faces, tempting and trapping us, 24/7. We are emotional eaters; instead of dealing with our feelings, any feelings, good or bad, we eat them. We eat to celebrate the good, and we eat to soothe the bad, and that is a sure path to excess weight gain.

"You can't control everything in life, but you can control what you put in your body."

How do you fix these problems? Easy, just act a little C.R.A.Z.Y.

Control your portions.

Reduce added sugars and highly processed foods.

Add proteins, carbs, and fats in balanced proportions.

Zero excuses. Zero deprivation. Zero eating your emotions.

YWhy? Find your WHY for weight loss and do it for YOU!

When you take control of your food, you take control of your health, and when you take control of your health, you gain control over your whole life. It's a trickle-down effect: you think more clearly, you're more productive, you feel better in your skin, more confident, more optimistic, and happier, and all those pluses affect those people around you in positive ways. Once you realize how strong you are by taking charge of your food and health, you can be strong in all aspects of your life—your career and ambitions, your personal finances, your relationships, you name it!

THE LOSE WEIGHT LIKE CRAZY PLAN
At A Glance

My plan is custom made for people like you who want to lose weight like crazy the smart way—without dieting. To help speed up weight loss and keep it off for good, it's important to combine portion-controlled nutrition with daily exercise; that's the scientifically established best way to drop pounds, tone your body, and become healthier fast. The plan in this book is a 30-day jump-start to a healthier life. But instead of thinking about the next 30 days, just start with today. Later, you can always advance to my *Ultimate Portion Fix* program and join my workouts on Beachbody On Demand to do more. See, this is about building healthy habits that become just a normal way of life. There is no expiration date on healthy living.

Your C.R.A.Z.Y. Cheat Sheet:

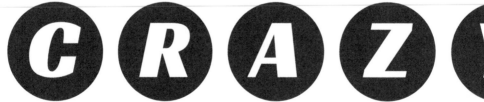

Control your portions.

Reduce added sugars and highly processed foods.

Add proteins, carbs, and fats in balanced proportions.

Zero excuses. Zero deprivation. Zero eating your emotions.

Y Why? Find your WHY for weight loss and do it for YOU.

The Details

Your Meals

Three satisfying meals per day and 2 snacks using my portion-control system.

Food Freedom: When you eat is up to you, and you can even spread out your food over more mealtimes, as long as you practice portion control.

Your Foods

You'll eat the rainbow:

- Vegetables
- Fruits
- Proteins like meats, fish, eggs, yogurt, and tofu.
- Carbohydrates like potatoes, rice, beans, whole-grain pasta and bread, even waffles.
- Healthy fats like avocado, almonds, and mozzarella cheese.
- Seeds & nuts; dressings
- Oils & nuts; nut butters
- Treats like cupcakes, cocktails, and chocolate as substitutions.

Your Drinks

Flat water (I'll show you how to figure out how many ounces per day is right for you).

- Sparkling water
- Coffee
- Tea
- Shakeology, Beachbody's nutrient-dense superfood protein shakes (one per day)
- Wine, beer, cocktails, as occasional treat substitutions.

Your Nutrients

You'll eat a balance of the 3 macronutrients in a healthy 40/30/30 split:

40% CARBOHYDRATES

30% LEAN PROTEINS

30% HEALTHY FATS

Don't worry: No math involved. My portion control system helps make the perfect mix automatic.

Your Clean Sweep

You'll cut out highly processed foods and sugars that contribute to weight gain and poor health and you'll learn the difference between real food and "food products." Again, all automatically.

Your Exercise

Work out on your terms, at home, when it's convenient for you. Shoot for 30 minutes of vigorous exercise per day. Brisk walking counts! But I've put together some fun full-body exercise routines for you to follow starting on page 236.

Your Truth Tribe

You'll check in regularly with a tribe of supporters for support and accountability.

(For plan details and instructions on getting started, see Part 2, on page 92.)

Part I

MY CRAZY LIFE

Why I Have No Business Being in the Business of Fitness and Nutrition

Let's be honest, I have no business being in the business of fitness and nutrition. If you look at the span of my crazy life, you would have never thought, "That girl is going to end up being a fitness and nutrition expert and a major influencer." After everything I've gone through, from physical injuries to emotional beatdowns, and never really being taught proper nutrition myself, how the hell did I end up here, and how can my experiences show you that you can lead a crazy healthy life, too? Well, let's dive in and find out.

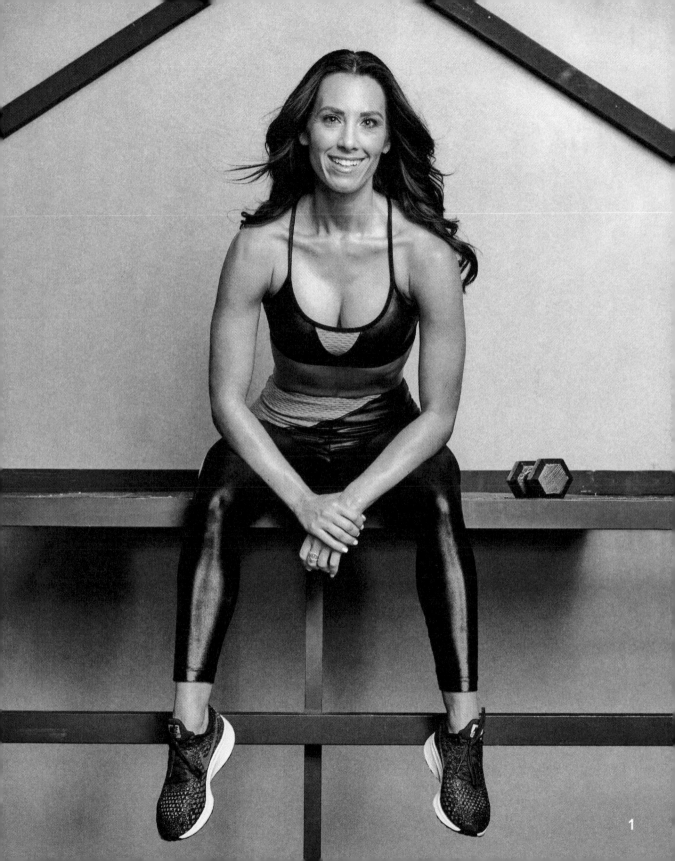

Chapter 1

BATTLING WEIGHT ISSUES AT EVERY SIZE

Commit to 30 days,
go all in, trust the process,
and watch what happens.

You don't have to be overweight to be out of shape, and you can be in great shape and still have weight to lose. This whole process of reaching an ideal, healthy weight and being fit can be very tricky. Learning to eat healthy can be incredibly hard, right? Right now, you're probably thinking, "Autumn, didn't you tell me eating healthy is easy? Eat my veggies, eat some fruit, watch my portion sizes, avoid overly processed foods. Now you're saying it's hard?!" Let me explain. Eating healthy IS easy, but we tend to overcomplicate it. If you haven't been taught the basic principles of good nutrition, if you're addicted to sugar or other highly processed foods, if you're not sure how to cook in a healthy way, or if you don't have a support system around you, then ya, eating healthy can be hard.

Let's go back to that part about overcomplicating it. This is a big one. We overcomplicate eating properly so much. It seems like every other day there's a new diet to follow. You open a magazine and it's talking about why you need to do some new cleanse. You turn on the TV and a talk show host is interviewing an expert about their new way of eating. There are a million different theories out there, so what do you do? You try one, then another, then you combine a little from this one and a little from that one and maybe add in something new from over here. Maybe something's working, but you're not sure exactly what component it is. Maybe it's not working, and maybe that's because you're not following any one specific plan completely. See how we overcomplicate it? That's what I'm here for. I'm here to unravel it all for you. I'm going to strip it down to a few basic principles that are proven to work. They haven't just worked for me, they've worked for hundreds of thousands if not millions of people who have followed my program, and now it's YOUR turn. In order for it to work, you'll need to go all in. You can't be wishy-washy, dipping your toe in this pool while also trying to dip a toe on the other foot in another pool. Give me 30 days, go all in, trust the process, and watch what happens. You're going to lose weight like CRAZY. But, before we dive into the plan, you might be wondering, "What makes her such an expert?"

Maybe you're thinking, "Look at this skinny woman. What does she know about needing to lose weight? I bet she's never struggled with it a day in her life."

Well, you're right and you're wrong. No, I've never had a significant amount of weight to lose, but that doesn't mean I haven't struggled with my weight or my body image. The first time I struggled with my weight was when I was 12 years old. I grew up in that small Italian neighborhood, I walked to and from school every day with my brother and sister, even in the snow. It wasn't uphill both ways, but we did walk the 4 blocks in both directions every day. I had recess at school every day, and when I got home and my homework was finished, I went outside to play. My cousins lived a block away. My grandparents lived 5 blocks away. There was a huge playground not too far from the building we owned and lived in, as well as a pool. Our building was also on a fairly big, gated lot, so I would also go outside and play in the lot for hours. The weekends were filled with bike riding and playing tag or hide-and-seek with all of my cousins at my grandparents' house on Sundays. The bottom line is, I never sat still.

It's a good thing I never sat still because my dad owned a pizza restaurant, and I grew up eating pizza, pasta, subs, New York–style cheesecake, chips and soda. A few nights a week my dad cooked a different dinner like beef stew, rainbow trout (one of my favorites), or meatloaf. But for the most part it was pizza, pasta, and subs. I don't remember eating vegetables very often, unless it was romaine or iceberg lettuce at my grandma's house on Sundays, and I'm sure we drank water but it doesn't stand out. It was mostly milk, soda, or juice. My high activity level and youth were combating my diet of carbs and sugar, but it was about to catch up with me.

I was a very skinny kid until I was about 12. Then I got hit with the trifecta that a lot of people experience: carb overload, insufficient exercise, and puberty! We moved from my little Italian neighborhood to the suburbs, and I could no longer just walk to my cousins' or grandparents' houses anymore. I took the bus to school, and there was no longer a huge yard to play in. I was also now in eighth grade, so the school workload was becoming more intense, meaning I was sitting way more, and last but not least, hormones! At 12, puberty set in, and I didn't have much information since I was being raised by a single dad, but hormones can come into play at any age, really.

So, here I was, this young girl that, up until this point, could eat anything she wanted, and did, and was still a twig. Out of nowhere I gained about 15 pounds. That might not sound like a lot, but it felt like a lot to me. My clothes didn't fit the same, I didn't have as much energy when I was dancing or playing, and I didn't feel great about myself. I was very aware that I was bigger than I had ever been, but I didn't understand why. I was a dancer, a competitive dancer. No one ever said anything to me about my size, but I knew that as a dancer I needed to be in better shape. I would look at fitness magazines and try to get tips from there on what I could do. I remember reading about the importance of being hydrated and that drinking water could help you lose weight. I was only 12 and I couldn't totally understand what I was reading, so I did the best I could to apply what I read in those magazines.

I remember thinking to myself one day, "OK, I'm doing this. I'm losing weight. I'm going to get in such great shape. People are going to be so impressed." I figured all I needed to do to lose weight was chug some water, so that's what I did. I remember I was watching TV, and I started with an 8-ounce glass of water. My goal was to finish it by the next commercial break, then I would refill during commercials and do it again. I did that for about an hour. My stomach was sloshing with water, and I had to pee every 5 seconds, but that was about it. I weighed myself the next morning. Nothing had changed, so in my mind drinking water wasn't going to work.

Then there were all those commercials on TV advertising a slimming shake. "Drink 2 shakes a day and eat one meal and you'll lose weight," they said. "OK, I'm going to do that," I thought. I had to save up the money to buy the shake, so I asked my dad if I could do some chores at the restaurant and get paid. He agreed, but he didn't know how I was planning on using it. After a few days, I saved up the money to buy the slimming shake. I walked to the drugstore down the street when no one was home, bought the chocolate flavor, and rushed home, ready to start my new plan. I hid the can of powder under some clothes in a dresser drawer in my room. I was so excited to make my first shake. I mixed the powder with some water and took a big swig, expecting it to be every bit as delicious as the pretty women in the commercials made it look. Ha, NO! It was disgusting. I almost spit it into the sink it was so bad! But I was determined to lose weight, so I took a few more sips. Nope, couldn't do it, it was just too gross. I went back to my room, and there I was, sitting on my bed with my can of gross slimming powder, so frustrated that I was back to square one. I was at a loss, I was 12 years old. How was I supposed to know what to do without someone to teach me? I gave up hope and continued with my mostly sedentary lifestyle except for my dance classes a few times a week, and I kept eating the way I had been eating because that's all there was in the house.

Two years later, I was in dance class. My teacher always gave us a little pep talk at the end of a lesson, and on this particular sunny, summer day she started talking about drugs. I think one of the older girls in class had asked her if she ever tried marijuana. She had all of us sit and she started to tell us a story about when she was in college. She was in college, but she was also dancing professionally. A friend of hers offered her marijuana, and she tried it. She went on to explain how she got the munchies after trying it, and that she ate an entire bag of chips. She tried it a few more times, and every time she had the munchies. She was eating foods like pizza and chips and drinking lots of soda, so she began to gain weight quickly, which was affecting her performance. When she realized she was gaining weight, she stopped using marijuana, and she stopped eating those unhealthy foods. This woman was my idol, so I took 2 things from that story that day: **1)** I was NEVER going to try drugs, ever, because drugs make you eat food that isn't good for you (I was only 14, I didn't think deeper into what she was saying) and **2)** chips and soda make you gain weight. That was the day I stopped drinking soda, but I didn't stop because she TOLD me to, I stopped because she SHOWED me how it had affected her life.

Eliminating soda had a huge impact on my body almost instantly. About 2 weeks after she gave us that talk, I walked into dance class in my jazz pants and a cropped T-shirt. I didn't really realize I had lost weight, but apparently everyone else did. As soon as I walked through the door everyone looked at me, and all the girls started to say how good I looked and asked me what I had been doing. My response was, "Nothing really, I stopped drinking soda 2 weeks ago?" Yes, I said it with a question mark on the end because what I was thinking was, "Did I really lose weight just from giving up soda?" When I got home after dance class, I got on the scale. Lo and behold, I was 5 pounds lighter. I couldn't believe it! It was so simple. Why hadn't anyone else told me this? I felt a little bit better about my body, but I was still carrying an extra 10 pounds. Giving up the soda helped and, for the time being, I was content with that small victory. It wasn't until six months later that I realized the true impact of my consistent, unhealthy food choices, lack of exercise, and carrying extra weight.

Crazy Soda Facts

About 40: Grams of sugar in a 12-ounce soda

51,100: Number of extra calories you would consume in a year if you drank one can of soda per day

3,500 calories equals approximately 1 pound of fat so that is an extra 14.6 pounds in a year from drinking one can of regular soda a day!

Over 470: Number of cans of soda the average American drinks per year

Coca-Colaproductfacts.com; Center for Science in the Public Interest; Diabetes Care

Drinking one soda a day **increases your risk of metabolic disease by 36%, and your risk of diabetes by 67%**

A soda a day may **increase triglycerides**, a blood fat that can lead to heart disease.

Get Rid of Soda

There are very few things that I'll tell you you can't have on my program, but soda is one of them. There are zero health benefits to it, and even the zero-calorie, zero-sugar ones are all highly processed, or laced with some version of "sugar" in order to taste sweet. It has no nutritional value and our body doesn't recognize it, so it can't tell how to use it, and it absolutely can lead to weight gain. Even worse, if you're drinking a lot of soda, you're probably not drinking enough water.

So, on the *Portion Fix* plan, soda is not approved. I understand that can be a challenge, and many of us are addicted to soda, so let's baby-step out of it. First, add up how much soda you're drinking in a day. Now, we're going to cut it in half. If you're drinking 30 ounces a day, cut it down to 15 ounces. Stay there for 3 days, then cut it in half again, so 8 ounces. Stay there for another 3 days, then halve it again to 4 ounces. Stay there for 3 more days, then cut out the soda completely. If you still need the caffeine, sub in a caffeinated tea or coffee, but the goal is not to over-caffeinate (more on this later).

HOW I DISCOVERED MY LOVE OF HEALTHY EATING AND FITNESS

I've mentioned that I had a crazy childhood, right?

My dad always encouraged us to be active, but neither my siblings nor I participated in your typical school sports. I danced, Bobby took karate, and Calie was on the high school crew team. My dad's favorite, and only form of exercise, was power walking. When I say power walking, I mean POWER WALKING. My dad could walk 5 miles in just under an hour. He had a route that he did through a park not far from our house. Pops was also big on us bonding as a family. One year when I was 7, he decided that on Thanksgiving Day we were going to walk from my grandma's house in Collinwood to dinner at my aunt's house in Mayfield Heights. How far is the walk, you ask? About 12 miles! This was the end of November in Cleveland, Ohio! It's freezing that time of year and usually snowing. But he insisted. We bundled up, packed a book bag of snacks, put our dog Crocket on the leash, and took off on foot at 7:00 a.m. My dad was the power walker, but we were kids. Bobby was 9 and Calie was 11. Let's not forget we were bundled up in snow gear, and because our route led us through the park where my dad did his regular power walks, that meant we had a steep hill to climb, too. I swear, I couldn't make this stuff up. I know it sounds crazy, and it was, but as I type this, I'm laughing thinking about that walk and the stories that we still tell about it.

We made that walk every Thanksgiving for 4 years. Even though I dreaded it, I could always do it no problem. In fact, I am a lot like my dad, I love to walk. If it was warm out, I probably would have loved it.

Once we moved to the suburbs, we stopped doing that tradition. That is until I was 14. We woke up on Thanksgiving morning that year, and my dad decided we were going to do our walk. It wasn't really safe to make the walk from our old neighborhood to my aunt's house anymore. Recession had hit Cleveland hard, and crime rates had skyrocketed in some areas. So, we were going to do it from our new house in the suburbs to my aunt's. Piece of cake, that was only about 5 miles. Except it wasn't a piece of cake. When we were making the walk when I was younger, I was also leading a much more active lifestyle. When we made the shorter walk this time, I had been living my sedentary, suburban life, and I was still carrying that extra 10 pounds, maybe even a little more on top of it. That 5-mile walk felt impossible. I was short of breath, and I struggled any time there was the slightest incline. I cried because I was uncomfortable in my own skin, and I just wanted to stop. At one point my dad looked over at me, a little in disbelief, and he asked, "What's wrong with you? You dance all the time." He wasn't being mean, he really didn't get why I was struggling so much and, honestly, neither did I. That walk was humbling. I was disappointed in myself. I was a little ashamed and even embarrassed. I was a competitive dancer; my body was supposed to be fit and strong. I wish I could say I quickly discovered the answers, but I didn't. It would be another 3 years before I began to learn and understand why my body wasn't as strong as it should have been. Why I felt so weighed down. Why I struggled to do something that should be so natural to all of us, walk.

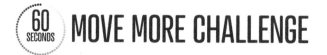

MOVE MORE CHALLENGE

Here are some simple ways to add more steps to your day that take just a minute:

- Park farther from your destination

- Use the stairs instead of the elevator

- Take a walk once a day

- Walk over to a coworker's desk instead of sending an email

Right before I turned 16, I moved to St. Louis to live with my mom. My dad had raised me, and he's an amazing father—I wouldn't trade that for the world—but he was strict, which was hard for someone who doesn't like being told what to do. But also, I was a young woman and I needed my mom for the woman stuff. My mom loved to exercise. She would put on her Jane Fonda VHS tapes or Denise Austin and follow along. I loved joining in. She also had a treadmill in her bedroom, in front of the TV, along with some hand weights. I still wanted to lose weight and feel better about my body, and I was still competing as a dancer. I was motivated, to say the least. That memory of barely being able to complete that 5-mile walk with my dad just a few years earlier still weighed on me, so I set a goal: I was going to be able to walk 5 miles without a struggle. I would get on the treadmill, set a moderate pace, and start walking. At first it was hard, and I would get bored really fast, so I started putting on music. I would tell myself, "You have to walk for 3 songs." After a few weeks I bumped it up to 4 songs, then 5. Then I would put on the TV, and I would tell myself, "Make it through one TV show and you'll have walked for 30 minutes." I did that several times a week until I was walking 3 to 5 miles on that treadmill without a problem. I was dancing 4 nights a week after school, as well. That's not all that changed, though. My mom cooked and ate very different than my dad. Obviously, my mom didn't own an Italian restaurant. We always had breakfast before school. I can't say my breakfast was healthy, even though I thought it was (I would eat a sleeve of graham crackers dipped in milk), but the milk at Mom's was skim, whereas Dad's was 2%, not a big difference, but a difference. When I lived with my dad, he would bring us hot lunch to school almost every day. It was either a sub sandwich with a bag of chips or a small pizza. At my mom's, I was responsible for packing my own lunch. The food options in the fridge were very different. There were tons of fruits and vegetables, wheat bread, not white bread, and cold cuts from the deli. My lunch was usually a sandwich, but sometimes I would put some veggies like sliced-up bell peppers or small broccoli florets on it, plus a piece of fruit and maybe a low-fat yogurt on the side. I wasn't drinking soda much anymore, so I drank water, a lot of water. We also always had a pretty healthy dinner. Things like grilled chicken, baked salmon, or steak. There was usually a carbohydrate side, and there was always a salad, and you had to eat salad. These salads were a little different than my grandma's back in Ohio. Although Grandma's salad was, and remains, the most delicious salad even if it wasn't the healthiest. My mom's salads were romaine and spinach with tomato and usually chopped-up bell pepper. I have to be honest, I didn't like veggies very much when I first moved in with my mom. I hadn't been eating them, so I hadn't developed a palate for them. I would always try what she had, though. I took baby steps with them. I would eat broccoli dipped in a little ranch dressing, carrot sticks, or cucumbers. I loved salad. It took me a while to start to like those damn bell peppers, though. But I have to say they are now one of my favorite veggies, and I'll often carry a whole pepper as a snack. I eat them just like apples!

All these changes were happening slowly, over the course of a few months. I wasn't focused on my weight much anymore. I noticed I had WAY more energy, and my clothes were fitting better. Without even trying, I had lost almost 20 pounds! I went from a size 8, sometimes 10, to a zero in a matter of months. I actually started wearing my mom's clothes for a little while because my clothes no longer fit. I finally felt comfortable in my own skin, I was light on my feet when I danced, and I had all the energy I needed.

This is where my love of healthy eating and fitness started. This showed me that I didn't have to diet to lose weight, I had to choose healthier options of the foods that I loved. I had to watch my portions, and I needed to move my body more than I had been. Simple. CRAZY simple.

60 SECONDS

YOU CAN DO ANYTHING FOR 60 SECONDS CHALLENGE

Pick an Exercise and Push Yourself.

Marching high-knees or jogging in place.

- Set a timer for 60 seconds and do one of these 2 exercises.

- See how many sets you can do in a day.

- Record your minutes and try to beat your total.

---

*CRAZY EASY, CRAZY POWERFUL **TIP #4***

Crowd Out the Bad with the Good

This is a practice I learned several years ago from the Integrative Institute of Nutrition. This journey is about taking small steps daily in the right direction. When you dive into the full *Portion Fix* program, you will see that you're going to be eating several servings of vegetables a day. For veggie lovers, like me, that's not a problem, but if you don't eat vegetables at all right now, going from none to 4 or 6 servings a day can feel like a lot. So, let's start small. If you don't like vegetables, don't worry, this can actually change once you start eating them regularly. A recent study from the University of Buffalo found that saliva contains proteins and those proteins can affect taste. Everything we eat is dissolved in saliva before hitting our taste receptor cells. What you eat dictates which proteins are expressed and present. With more exposure, your taste can eventually change. Is your mind blown like mine was?! That's great news. You really can learn to like veggies.

Another study shows that you need to be exposed to a food up to 7 times before you might start to like that food, so be patient. If at first you don't succeed, try and try again.

Pick 1 or 2 new vegetables to try every few days. Try having the vegetable prepared a few different ways. Let's take broccoli, for instance: You can have it raw in a salad, sautéed with a little olive oil, garlic and sea salt, grilled or even baked. If you're looking for delicious ways to season your vegetables, check out my cooking show *FIXATE*, found on the online streaming service Beachbody On Demand. You'll also find many different ways to prepare your vegetables on the cooking show. The key is to start trying them. As you find veggies that you like, write them down and add them to your veggie arsenal, which will automatically "crowd out" the unhealthy foods in your diet. This way, by the time you start doing the full program, you'll be ready.

All of this is to say, it's the same for you. You don't have to do a complete 180 on your nutrition today. You can make small changes. You can follow the baby steps that I'm giving throughout the book, if that's the pace that works for you. Or, you can go all-in and follow the *Portion Fix* program as I have it written in Part 2 of this book. Either way you're going to lose weight like crazy. The only difference will be how fast. The healthier you eat and the more you move, the faster you will lose.

The Final Straw

The last time I battled with my weight I was 26 and had just moved to LA. Once I lost weight living with my mom, I was able to maintain my weight fairly easily. I fluctuated between 95 and

104 pounds from my junior year in high school until my junior year in college. When I was in college, my eating habits went to hell. I was a broke college student. I didn't have the stocked refrigerator from Whole Foods that I had living with my mom. I waited tables at a Mexican restaurant, so I either ate there or at the school cafeteria. I was still young, so I had that working for me. I was also a dance major, dancing 4 to 6 hours a day. Plus, I waited tables most nights of the week, so I was on my feet for an 8-hour shift, and did I mention I liked to dance? When I got home from work, I'd get cleaned up and head out to a club with friends to dance the night away. Moving my body that much kept the weight off, so I didn't think twice about my crappy eating habits. But as soon as I left school, those eating habits caught up with me. I gained 10 pounds, it didn't make me obese by any stretch but on my frame and in my mind that was not good. Not that big of a deal, once again, I wasn't comfortable in my clothes or my skin.

I was living in LA by myself and waiting tables at a popular restaurant known for its huge portions and its cheesecake (always with the cheesecake). I was no longer dancing (you'll find out why in the next part of this book) and since I was new in town, I didn't have many friends, so I wasn't going out. I went from being very active to once again being fairly sedentary, so I decided to join a gym. I was going 4 to 5 days a week for 30 minutes, doing mostly steady-state cardio on the treadmill or elliptical. I wasn't gaining any more weight, but I also wasn't losing any. That's when I met my future husband, and you guessed it, bring on the new relationship habits! Lots of dinners out, cocktails and wine and late-night eating, since we both worked in the restaurant industry and didn't get off work until midnight most nights. We would come home from work, crack open a bottle of wine, put out the cheese, crackers, and salami, and watch TV together. The scale started to move but not in the direction I wanted it to. I gained another 3 or 4 pounds.

At this point, I was also looking for a talent agent. I had a meeting with one in particular that I was excited about, and I brought my headshots, which he seemed to really like. We had a great conversation about my background in dance and the acting classes I was taking. At the end of the meeting, he said he was looking forward to working with me, there was just one thing. "How much do you weigh?" he asked. A wave of terror came over me. I didn't want to say my real weight. I was around 118 pounds, and I know that is not a big number, but you have to remember it's all relative. For my body and my build, I was 15 or 20 pounds heavier than normal. I told him I weighed around 110 or 112 pounds. Then he said something that shocked me. "OK, I need you to get down to around 103 to 105 pounds. Do you think you can do that? Casting directors really want leading women to be small, just look at Courtney Cox." I said I could do that no problem, but what I was really thinking was, "Houston, we have a problem! A HUGE problem!" I had been trying to lose weight for the last year with no luck. Now I was being told I couldn't be signed until I was down to 105 pounds! Once again, I was disappointed in my body. I felt like I wasn't good enough because of my weight. I was a young woman, trying to find my way in a very challenging, judgmental business and I was being asked to do something I knew my body couldn't or really shouldn't do.

I was so mad when I got home. I told my boyfriend what the talent agent had said, and he joked, "He wants you to get down to a buck-five?!" I was annoyed that he didn't think I could do it, so I was more determined than ever. I even bet him 20 dollars that I could do it in the next 2 months. I lost that bet. I kept working out, but my eating habits didn't change. No amount of exercise was going to out-train my bad diet. I never signed with that talent agent. In fact, the only time I've been back down to 105 pounds in the last 15 years was the day I took the stage for my first fitness competition, 8 years after that talent agent asked me to do it. I was carb depleted, dehydrated, and had been working out 2 to 3 hours a day for months. My body is not meant to weigh 105 pounds anymore.

By the time we got married, two years later, I weighed a comfortable 112 pounds. But in the back of my mind I had that number from college in my head that I was trying to achieve. Y'all can we please keep in mind that in college we are still growing and changing into adults?! You're not necessarily supposed to weigh at 28 years old what you weighed at 18 years old. We need to reframe our expectations. We need to focus on health, instead of that number on the scale. It took me a long time to learn that. The scale is just one form of measurement. For this story we will continue to use it but I can't emphasize enough the importance of focusing on being the healthiest version of yourself. You are not a number on the scale.

It wasn't until I became a personal trainer, got married, and got pregnant with my son that I decided to learn about nutrition. I wanted to know what I needed to fuel my body for my growing baby, so I started to study and learned the difference between calories in a protein, a carbohydrate, and a fat. I started to learn more about the importance of vegetables and lean proteins. I began to read labels and realized the "healthy" breakfast cereal I was eating every morning was LOADED with sugar.

I studied all throughout my pregnancy, and when I had my son, I had set a goal for myself: I had read over and over again in the tabloid magazines about all these celebrities having babies and how fast they were losing their baby weight. On average they were losing it in 3 to 4 months. I had also read a statistic that said something along the lines of, for every month you keep baby weight on, after the first year, it becomes significantly harder to get it off. I'm paraphrasing that because I don't remember the exact wording, but whatever it was, I knew that wasn't going to be me. I was going to lose all of my baby weight in 4 months. I was a personal trainer. I had a specialty in pre- AND post-natal fitness. I had been learning all about nutrition. If a celebrity could do it, so could I. I didn't have a chef. I didn't have a trainer. I didn't have a nanny to help take care of Dominic. What I had was my work ethic and my goal. I put one thought in my head about food. Because I was breastfeeding, everything I ate, my son would eat, too. If I wouldn't feed it to him, then I couldn't feed it to myself.

I had to have an emergency C-section with Dominic, so that put me behind the eight ball with my goal. I couldn't exercise or even walk much for 6 weeks. That meant I had to be even more diligent about my nutrition. I didn't cut calories—I couldn't because I was breastfeeding—I didn't deprive myself, I just made small changes. I gave up my sugar-packed cereal in favor of eggs, whole-wheat toast, and sometimes veggies for breakfast. I cut way back on the amount of sugar I put in my morning coffee. I stopped eating granola bars 2 to 3 times a day as a "healthy snack" and instead ate fruit or veggies. I started cooking healthier dinners, and I only drank water. After I was cleared to begin light exercise, I started taking Dominic on 2 walks a day. I would put him in the stroller, and we would go for a 3-mile walk after breakfast. I didn't really plan it to be 3 miles, I just walked because it felt good to get outside and move. I would take another walk in the late afternoon before we began our bedtime routine. If the weather was bad, I would walk on the used treadmill I had saved to purchase. If Dominic was on the floor doing tummy time, I would get down and do crunches or hold a plank. I fit in what I could, when I could. I gained 36 pounds during my pregnancy; I weighed in at 148 when I checked into the hospital to give birth. I lost all 36 pounds plus 3 more for a total of 39 pounds in 3 months and 4 days. I hit my goal 3 days early, weighing 109 pounds, and I've maintained that weight for the last 11 years.

I wasn't perfect, there were good days and hard days. There were times where the scale didn't budge, and I felt like it was hopeless. I celebrated the small victories, and I cried when I was frustrated, but ultimately, I trusted the process and the path that I was on. It will be the same for you. I don't expect you to be perfect. I'm not asking you to be. No one is perfect; we aim for progress not perfection on Team AC. You will have good days, and you will have hard days. They are all part of this process. But, here's the cool part, you don't fail unless you quit. There's no timeline on this. Had I not reached my goal in 4 months, I wouldn't have given up. I would have celebrated how far I'd come and kept going. I'll say it again, this isn't about being perfect, this is about making progress, striving to be a LITTLE better today than you were yesterday. To learn a little bit more about yourself, to work toward leading the healthiest life possible, whatever that looks like and means for you, that's what we're going to discover together.

AUTUMN'S ATTITUDE **ADJUSTMENT**

Choose Your Hard

It can be hard to choose healthy foods over junk foods more often than not. It can be hard to stop emotionally eating and start eating to fuel your body. It's hard to make time for your workout every day. It's hard to burn and sweat and be out of breath. It's also hard to be uncomfortable in your own skin. It's hard to feel bad physically, mentally, and emotionally. It's hard to look in the mirror and not recognize yourself. The difference is, by choosing the hard of health, by choosing to work out, eat right and practice self-care, ALL the other stuff goes away. You feel strong, proud, and confident in who you are. So, choose your hard.

Change Up Your Coffee Order

Let's talk about coffee: I love it as much as the next person.
I enjoy starting my day with a hot cup, not because I need it but
because I really like the taste of it. But there is a difference
between coffee and coffee beverages. What do I mean? Well
coffee is just that, coffee or espresso, black. Coffee beverages are
the ones that are loaded with sugar and cream. Or the ones you
get at the coffee house that are huge, with several pumps of sweet
syrup, topped with whipped cream, caramel sauce, chocolate sauce,
sprinkles, and more. That's not coffee, that's a coffee-flavored
beverage. Some of those drinks pack well over 1,000 calories
and loads of sugar, more than you should even consume in
the day.

So, when it comes to coffee, let's take it back to the basics.
Coffee or espresso with 1 teaspoon of organic raw sugar or stevia,
and if you prefer, you can do a dash of cream, or milk. By dash,
I mean 1 to 2 tablespoons at most. I used to drink coffee with
several packets of sugar, plus flavored creamer; it took a while
to break the habit. I had to start slow. I went from 2 packets of
Sweet'N Low to 1½ packets, to 1 packet, then to a ½ of a packet,
then I switched to organic sugar in the raw and just used 1 packet.
I went from a lot of flavored creamer to a little less, then just a
dash, then I stopped buying it and switched to no creamer at all.
Now, if I want a little creaminess to my coffee, I'll do a splash
of unsweetened coconut milk.

I made this switch 10 years ago. It took me several weeks to
cut out all that extra sugar, but once I did, I felt so much better, and
I still enjoy the taste of my coffee. If you're drinking sweet coffee
beverages every day, start to take small steps to cut back. Not only
will it help your waistline, it will help your wallet as well.

"I lost 117 pounds . . . Now I'm lean, healthy and I'm STRONG!"

—**Hannah D.**, 31, Independent Team Beachbody Coach, Machesney Park, IL

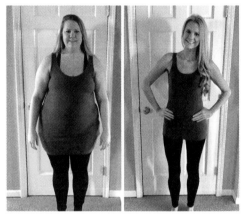

Day 1: 237 lbs.   Day 354*: 120 lbs.

Over the course of eight years, Hannah D. gained 115 pounds topping 237 pounds, and her health deteriorated. She suffered from extreme fatigue, joint pain, foggy brain, high blood pressure, gastrointestinal issues, and hair loss.

"I would look in the mirror and not recognize myself," Hannah says. "I was depressed about my weight and I felt so insecure that I didn't want to go places where people would see me." When taking family pictures she would try to hide behind her kids and husband. She was heartbroken, feeling that she couldn't be the best mom her family deserved. She tried all sorts of diets and exercise programs, but nothing worked. "I felt really lost and discouraged," she says.

What changed? Hannah started my *21 Day Fix* program and found that it solved her biggest food-related problem: portion control.

She also was surprised to learn that she could actually do the modified 30-minute at-home workouts. "I was someone who couldn't even do a single jumping jack in the beginning," says Hannah, "so if I can do it, ANYONE CAN DO IT!"

In 2018, Hannah weighed 237 pounds. Now she's a trim, healthy 120! "I've never been strong," she says, "and now I'm lean, healthy and I'm STRONG. I feel amazing! I'm so confident in who I am now, from the inside out!"

Chapter 2

OVERCOMING PHYSICAL SETBACKS

Let's get out from behind the eight ball.

I was 5 years old in kindergarten. My parents had already been divorced for 3 years. My dad had a house in Euclid, Ohio that we stayed at when we were with him, and my mom had an apartment that wasn't too far away. I don't really have any memories of my mom's place. I only remember one day in that apartment, there are no other memories of it except that one fateful day. My mom had my sister, brother and me for her days of the week. We had been at the apartment playing all day. It was a 2-bedroom, and my siblings and I shared a bedroom on one side of the apartment, while my mom's room was on the other side. Bobby and I had been running back and forth chasing each other, and as we were running, my hip started to hurt. I remember stopping multiple times and saying to my mom, "Mom, my hip hurts." Not much was made of it since I kept playing, but over the course of the night it continued to feel sore. That night I went to sleep with my brother and sister in the double bed we shared—actually, Bobby had his own single, but he always came and slept with us after my mom left the room. In the middle of the night, the pain in my hip woke me up, and I tried to get out of bed, but I collapsed as soon as I put weight on my legs. My mom heard me fall and rushed to the room to see what happened. She thought I'd fallen out of bed—something that actually happened fairly often since there were 3 of us, and that didn't leave a lot of room to roll over in your sleep.

My mom carried me back to her room, and I went back to sleep. A few hours later the alarm went off. It was time to get up for school, but when I rolled over, again a shooting pain went through my hip. At 5, I couldn't very well articulate the feeling, so I just repeated my previous complaint, "Mom, my hip hurts." I think she thought I was faking to try to get out of going to school, but I was in serious pain. Frustrated and in a rush to get 3 kids ready for school, my mom just said, "Autumn, get up!" I knew she meant business, so I tried to get out of bed. But once again, I collapsed in a heap, this time SCREAMING in pain. In that instant my mom knew something was seriously wrong. I laid there on the floor sobbing, not able to stand or even really move. My mom quickly called my dad. Even though they had a tumultuous relationship, she knew this was no time for fighting. She told my dad she was rushing me to the E.R. My dad said he would meet us there. Into the car we went, I had to be carried, and I laid across the back seat because I couldn't even sit up from the pain. I don't remember the car ride to the hospital, but I remember arriving. Doctors met us outside and helped lift me out of the car. They tried to sit me in a wheelchair, but again the pain shot through my hip like a hot knife and I screamed. At this point my dad had arrived. He picked me up and carried me into the hospital. Instantly I was surrounded by doctors and nurses. The details are foggy after that, but they are there in my mind like shadows, snippets of a dream half-remembered. Test after test, was run, with no answers. At one point the doctors thought I might have a flesh-eating bacterium consuming my hip from the inside— I'm glad I was too young to understand it all, but my parents were visibly terrified, and that I understood. There was a massive needle coming toward my little body (they were going to draw fluid from my hip), and my mom threw her body on top of mine. The doctors and nurses dragged her out of the room screaming while my dad held me down on the table. That test came back negative, too.

Tons of tests were run over the course of several days, and all of them came back inconclusive. I was in the hospital for a week; the upside was it was Christmastime, so Santa was making his way around the facilities, delivering toys to all of the kids. My family was also coming to visit, bringing lots of coloring books and crayons, and I got to watch a lot of cartoons. But ultimately, my weeklong stay at Rainbow Babies & Children's Hospital in Cleveland, Ohio, turned up no answers as to why I had such unbearable pain in my hip. I was sent home on crutches. My parents were told I may never walk again, and that they needed to be very careful of the activities I participated in. Since they didn't know what was wrong or what caused it, they didn't know what could possibly retrigger the injury. After a few weeks at home my hip got better. I was off the crutches and back to being a normal kid. BUT, and this is a big but, my parents were very leery for several years about letting me participate in any extracurricular activities. This was the first of many setbacks in my life. The first of many that would put me behind the eight ball.

You see, even at 5, I knew I wanted to dance. In fact, it's a running joke in my family that I came out of the womb dancing, since my mom never actually made it to the delivery room with me. She had me in the labor room. According to my dad, I shot out like a football. I wasn't waiting for anyone; when I was ready, I made my appearance into the world. So ya, I wanted to dance from a very young age. But the doctors had warned my parents about my hip, so at 5 years old, when I begged them to sign me up for dance classes, the answer was no. At 6, 7, and 8, the answer was no. I took my first dance class in eighth grade, when I was 13 years old. After years of begging, my dad finally realized my hip was no longer a threat, and I was able to enroll at Spotlight Dance Center, in Mayfield Heights, Ohio.

I had some of the best teachers in my life at that school, but I'll get to that later. I wanted to be a competitive dancer; there was just one problem. All the girls on the competition dance team had been dancing for years. When I say years, I mean they had at least 5 if not 6 years of experience on me. How was I going to get on this team that I wanted to be a part of so bad when I was so far behind the eight ball? I was going to work my ass off, that's how.

I was going to practice and practice and practice. I never missed a class. In fact, when I was sick, I would lie and tell my dad I felt fine, and even go to school, just so I wouldn't have to miss dance class. I asked my teacher what I could do to get better or to be more involved with the studio, and after a few months she let me come to help with the younger classes. I didn't get paid; I didn't get a discount on my lessons; I was in it to learn and to be the best version of me. Two years into dancing at Spotlight, I made the competition team! This was a valuable lesson for me. This was the first time I saw that talent will get you so far, but heart and perseverance will get you the rest of the way. I never was and never will be the most technical dancer in a room, but you'll be hard-pressed to find someone with more passion or a stronger work ethic than me.

And that's the point, with this program, as with anything in life: It takes dedication, it takes perseverance. Others might be stronger than you, have more endurance or less weight to lose, but if you have the drive and commitment, eventually, you'll be the one pulling ahead, even if you started behind the eight ball.

AUTUMN'S ATTITUDE ADJUSTMENT

You're Not ALWAYS Going to Be Motivated, So Learn to Be Disciplined

One of the first questions I'm always asked when being interviewed about my fitness routine is, "How do you stay so motivated?" Answer: I'm not always motivated, but I AM always disciplined. There are days I'm feeling it and days that I'm not. The days I'm not feeling it are the days I push even harder because that's how you make progress, that's how you become mentally stronger, that's how you prove to yourself that you can do hard things. You won't always be motivated, so learn to be disciplined. Discipline is something I learned at a young age. It's a part of the dance culture, especially if you're on the competition team. Everyone is required to take ballet, even if you don't compete in it. That way you're always working on technique. Pink tights, black leotard, black ballet skirt, hair pulled back in a bun, that's how you show up to ballet class. You practice, you work, you keep going, even when you're tired, even when you've done it 50 times already. You don't practice until you get it right, you practice until you can't get it wrong. That's discipline.

So yeah, I learned it at a young age. Others might just be learning it as an adult. It applies in all areas of life, including nutrition. I'm not always motivated to eat well, I have days I want to have a few more glasses of wine than I should, or I want to sit on the couch, drown out the day, and eat ice cream from the tub, but I don't do that because I'm disciplined about taking care of my body for my health. Instead, I enjoy the 1 to 2 glasses of wine that I'm allowed, or the few scoops of ice cream instead of the pint. I don't deprive myself, but I don't overindulge either. That's discipline.

Physical setbacks and limitations can definitely make something harder, but nothing is impossible. Impossible, a word that tries to break you, but instead of letting it break us, let's break impossible into, I'm-possible. YOU are an infinite possibility. You can do anything you set your heart and mind to. It might come easier for some than others, but if you put in the work you can achieve the goal. We have the Paralympics; these are competitive games at the highest level for people with physical limitations. They are showing us every day what can be achieved. I follow some of the most inspiring athletes on social media, vets who no longer have their legs and are still in incredible shape, doing pull-ups in their wheelchair. We see people make miraculous recoveries after terrible accidents. This doesn't just happen; this happens because they are dedicated to making it happen. They believe in themselves; they believe so much that they CAN do it, that they DO do it.

Let me ask you this, HOW BAD DO YOU WANT IT? If you have ever done one of my workout programs, you know this is something I will shout in the middle of a workout when I'm pushing you to your limits. I don't shout it just because it sounds fun or gets a crowd going at a live workout. I shout it to remind you of what you are working toward. Is your goal to lose weight like crazy? Is your goal to live a healthy life no matter how crazy life gets? If the answer is yes, then I'm going to ask you again, HOW BAD DO YOU WANT IT?! Do you feel it in your soul? Do you believe it's possible? Are you ready to put in the work? Change doesn't come easy. Are you willing to make some sacrifices? Are you willing to sweat? Are you willing to do things you've never done to have the healthy body you've always wanted? Are you ready to trust me completely to take you on this journey and help you lose weight like CRAZY, even if you have a crazy life? If you said yes, GREAT! Let's get started.

CRAZY EASY, CRAZY POWERFUL TIP #6

Begin with Breakfast

Breakfast is known as the most important meal of the day. This may bring up a lot of debate. Maybe you've read about the recent research questioning the importance of breakfast. That research, published in *BMJ* (*British Medical Journal*) in 2019, analyzed 13 breakfast studies and found that skipping breakfast doesn't lead to weight gain and eating breakfast isn't an effective way to lose weight. But other earlier studies have shown that people who regularly eat breakfast tend to weigh less than people who don't eat it. Who to believe? Well, you can experiment for yourself. Try eating breakfast every day. I'm not familiar with any studies showing that eating breakfast makes you gain weight. What I do know from my personal experience and my clients' is that putting fuel into your tank within 1 hour of waking can help boost your metabolism and keep you from overeating later on.

If you take the word "breakfast" and break it into 2 words, what do you get? BREAK, FAST. That is what you are doing. You are breaking the fast that just occurred while you slept. You've likely gone at least 10 hours, maybe more, without eating, so now it's time to put some fuel in to start your day. If you're not a big breakfast person that's OK, it doesn't have to be a lot of food. It can be something as simple as a piece of fruit or some plain Greek yogurt. If you're anything like me, and you love breakfast, feel free to make it a bigger meal, but beware of overly processed foods. Stick to foods that are as close to WHOLE FOODS as possible. My favorite breakfast is steel-cut oats flavored with a dash of cinnamon, vanilla extract, and ½ teaspoon of maple syrup, along with turkey breakfast sausage and sautéed broccoli. You can also check out the breakfast recipes in the back of this book.

Things to avoid when picking your breakfast foods are the super sugary foods. I'm talking about store-bought muffins and pastries, cereal with more than 8 grams of sugar per serving, white breads and milkshakes disguised as coffee drinks.

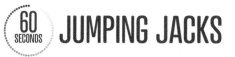

60 SECONDS JUMPING JACKS

Start with 60 seconds of jumping jacks, followed by
a 30-second rest, then jog in place for 60-seconds.

- See how many times throughout the day you can do this
  2-set challenge.

- Record your results and try to better them!

A Setback Can
Lead to an Even Better
Come Back

Being 5 years old and dealing with my hip injury was the
first time I had to overcome a physical setback, but it definitely
wasn't the last. I had plenty of ankle sprains over the years, a mild
concussion from being dropped during a lift in a dance rehearsal,
2 car accidents (neither time was I the driver), and plenty of bumps
and bruises over the years. My body was going through it before
I ever even got to college. The next big physical obstacle came my
junior year in college. I was a dance major at a small performing
arts school in St. Louis. I was taking a pretty big emotional beating
from my ballet master, which was wearing me down. I had already
taken one semester off to participate in the Disney College Program,
it was a much-needed break, but my instructors looked at it as
a lack of dedication.

There's pushing someone to be the best version they can be,

and then there's pushing someone past what their body is actually physically capable of doing, and that can lead to injury. I was being pushed past what my body could actually, physically do. Remember, I started dancing 7 years later than most girls. This has a huge impact on your body mechanics. When you are young, your bones have not fully hardened. That means you have an easier time working certain positions that might not come so naturally the older you get. Turnout is one of them. My turnout is terrible for a dancer. Turnout is where you turn your toes out 180 degrees, but you do this from the hips, not the ankles. When you start practicing this at a young age, it's easier to work into a better turnout, but when you start it at 13, it's not so easy. Then there are genetics, which also probably didn't help me. I had been dancing for 8 years at this point, dancing through sprained ankles, pushing my hips past what they could do, working my flexibility further than what my spine wanted. All of it was starting to take a toll on my body. My back and my knees hurt on a regular basis. I would feel it when I arched backward, I would feel it when I stretched my legs, and I would really feel it when I jumped. By the middle of my junior year I was dancing through some pretty serious pain. I did not have a good relationship with my ballet master (also a story to come later) but bottom line, I was getting no sympathy from him. In fact, when I would hold back in class due to the pain, he would pick on me that much more. I remember leaving ballet class one day and walking back to my apartment with a bit of a limp. My roommate asked me, "What's wrong?"

My eyes started to well up with tears, the pain was so intense. I said, "It feels like there's a searing hot poker in my spine."

She gave me a look of concern but didn't really know what to say. Just as we opened our apartment door, I sneezed and instantly buckled to the floor. The pain was so bad it took the wind out of me. I laid there crying; I couldn't move. I knew it was time to see a doctor.

It took a few days before I could really even move. I skipped classes, which didn't go over well, but I couldn't move more than to go from my bed to the couch. A week later I had an appointment with my doctor. The news wasn't good. My hips were uneven, my right leg was slightly longer than my left, I had a mild case of scoliosis and, oh ya, a bulging disc in my lower spine. Talk about a body not built to dance. This was a crushing blow. What the doctor said next was even worse: "If you keep dancing as much as you are, there's a good chance you will end up needing back surgery before you're 21. If you stop now, you can lead a completely normal life with no real issues." In an instant, everything I had been working for was taken away from me. Back surgery wasn't an option. That meant giving up my dream of becoming a professional dancer. The physical injuries combined with the emotional trauma I was experiencing at school (more on that later) had taken their toll. I left my performing arts college one semester shy of graduating. It honestly felt like it was the end of the world for me. I had no idea what I was going to do with my life if I didn't dance. But you know what? The universe has a funny way of giving you exactly what you need, even if you don't know you need it.

I thought I wanted to be a professional dancer. I spent the first half of my life dedicated to that dream. But having that dream taken away from me actually led me to a passion I didn't even know I had. It led me to a career I didn't even know I wanted. It wasn't until I had moved to LA, spent 2 years as a waitress (although I had already been waiting tables for years before that) and 4 months as a casting director's assistant, sitting at a desk 10 to 12 hours a day that the idea of fitness came to mind. I knew I couldn't take much more sitting at that desk. I was bored out of my mind, even though it was an incredibly busy office. I started to think about other jobs that I could do. I didn't want to go back to waiting tables—the money was good but unpredictable. My friend suggested being a dance instructor. I thought about it, but I just couldn't do it. I couldn't even bring myself to take a dance class due to the lack of confidence I had from what I experienced in college. How could I teach others to dance? Not only did I not have faith in my ability to teach, it was too personal. I was still devastated that I couldn't dance professionally, and if I was ever going to dance again, it was going to be for me.

But my friend's suggestion sparked another idea: I started researching what it would take to be a personal trainer, what types of jobs I could have, the type of people I could help and what education I needed. I had 9 years of dance training. As a dance major, I had taken anatomy classes, so I was very familiar with body mechanics. I was also a stickler for form, since that had been drilled into me over the years. I found the most reputable certification there was, the personal training certification through the National Academy of Sports Medicine. If I was going to do it, I was going to do it right. I was going to get the best education

I could, shy of going back to school. I studied for that exam for 4 months. I knew the book like the back of my hand. I went to the live trainings, and when the day came to take my test, I crushed it. I was a certified personal trainer!

I've been a trainer for more than 15 years now. I've held multiple different certifications, not just from NASM but from ACE (American Council on Exercise), AFPA (American Fitness Professionals Association), and AFAA (Athletics and Fitness Association of America). I even have a specialty in pre- and postnatal fitness. After spending years as a trainer, I wanted to expand my knowledge so I could be more well-rounded. I began to study nutrition. I devoured everything I could about how food impacts your body. I eventually went through a yearlong course, through the Integrative Institute of Nutrition, and have even taken advanced courses in gut health. Teaching people how to exercise properly, making it fun, showing you that you can do hard things, making nutrition accessible to everyone, and teaching you how to eat in a way that fuels your body without depriving your body is my passion. I am living THAT dream. I could have let my injuries and physical limitations stop me from being active. I could have used them as an excuse to become inactive, but instead I let them motivate me. I let them teach me who I was and who I wanted to be. I hope that I can share what I've learned with you to help you lose weight like crazy and live a crazy, healthy life no matter what your circumstances!

Taking Care of
Your Body Can Help Heal
Your Body Faster

It was the summer of 2017; I had been a Super Trainer with Beachbody for almost 6 years. I had finished development on my fifth program, *80 Day Obsession*. We were just shy of a month away from going into filming. This was a big deal! I would be filming the program in real time. That means I would be showing up on set every day for 80 days. That's 13 weeks of filming. No one had ever done it, not just with Beachbody, anywhere. I would be the first trainer in history to film a workout program in real time. This might not sound that hard, but believe me, it's a task of gigantic proportions. I couldn't get sick, I couldn't get injured, I'd have to show up no matter what, sore muscles, tired, feeling bloated, cramps, not in the mood, didn't matter. If you don't know me, allow me to introduce myself. I'm Autumn Calabrese, and I LOVE a challenge and getting to be the first! Oh my gosh, you better believe I'm going to rise to that challenge. I was on cloud nine, proud of the program I designed, crazy-happy about my cast, and ready to do the damn thing.

My schedule was intense. I had a week of rehearsals, a week-long vacation, another week of rehearsals, and then our biggest event of the year, Beachbody Summit. The first week of rehearsals went great. I left for vacation feeling good. I had a great time in Hawaii with my son and family and came back ready to get back to

work. We jumped back into rehearsals, running 2 workouts
a day, full speed, no compromises. That's 2 hours of working out,
which shouldn't be a problem for me at all. Just as we were wrapping
up the last workout, I felt something in my hip catch. "Damn that
hurts," I said. My fitness director asked what hurt, and I explained
that I tweaked my hip. I didn't think much of it. I stretched and
went home. As the night went on, I knew I was in trouble. I just
didn't realize how much trouble. By the time I woke up the next
morning, I could barely walk. The pain in my hip was excruciating.
I've dealt with my back going out multiple times over the years.
When it does, I know how to take care of it. I'm usually out of
commission for about 10 days, and then I need to ease back in.
This pain was different. This pain brought back memories of that
5-year-old girl not being able to walk. As a fitness professional,
I have a team of experts I can call on to help me when I'm injured.
I rallied the troops. I had my structural integration specialist at
my house for a 2-hour session. She started to work on me and said
she had never seen my body in that condition. I cried through
the entire session from the pain. The next day I went and saw my
physical therapist. He had the same opinion; he had never seen
me this bad before. I was leaving the next day for a big Beachbody
fitness conference in New Orleans called "Summit." I survived
the plane ride by sitting on a tennis ball, allowing it to dig into my
gluteus maximus to relieve some of the pain in my sciatic nerve.
I enlisted my friends (who are also Beachbody coaches) to join me
onstage for my workouts. I couldn't let anyone know just how
bad it was. You see, we were scheduled to start filming a week after
Summit. If my CEO found out how bad I was hurting, he might

postpone the filming, or worse, change the way we were going to film the program all together. If I wasn't onstage or at an event at Summit, I was working with an amazing acupuncturist that I found there in New Orleans. I was getting just enough relief to get by. Through all of this a few thoughts kept running through my mind: "This isn't getting better in the normal time frame. Is it going to get better? What if it doesn't? Is my career over? I have to film in a week, I can't work out, I need my body to be on point, even on day one, shit, shit, shit!" I had already been eating pretty clean, since I was going to be filming in a few weeks, but when I realized I was injured and wouldn't be able to work out leading up to the filming, I dialed my nutrition in that much more. I implemented every principle I know, not only to keep me in tip-top shape, but to help my body recover faster.

Everything you eat you become. Think about that: Every single thing that you put into your body is what your body becomes. What you eat fuels your body, it helps your cells repair and rejuvenate. What you eat determines how quickly you eliminate waste, if your tissue is inflamed or not, which genes express themselves and which ones don't. I followed all of the principles I've created for *Portion Fix*, all of the principles I'm going to teach you in this book. It took me 3 weeks to recover from that hip injury. It turns out, I had sprained my entire hip complex, but I'm proud to say, I showed up on day one of filming looking and feeling my absolute best. That wouldn't have been possible without proper nutrition. I also showed up every single day for 13 weeks to film *80 Day Obsession*. My cast followed my nutrition principles as well, and you know what? Not one person was sick in 13 weeks, not one person got injured, everyone filmed every single day of that workout, and everyone got shredded. Now it's your turn!

You Are What You Eat

So don't be fast, easy, cheap, or fake. It's time to start thinking about food for what it truly is—fuel for your body. When you look at it through this lens, it becomes much easier to make healthy choices. When you are deciding what to eat, ask yourself this one question: "Is this the best possible option to fuel my body for the results that I want?" If the answer is no, move on to something else that is a good fuel source. I'm not saying you can't ever have a treat or that you have to restrict yourself. In fact, my plan is the exact opposite. But, I do want you to start looking at food in a different light, from a perspective that makes it easier to make healthy choices the majority of the time.

*CRAZY EASY, CRAZY POWERFUL **TIP #7***

Take Out the Trash

It's very hard to eat well when you're surrounded by junk, so let's get rid of it. This might feel challenging; we can have a strong emotional attachment to food. For some, you might have a hard time "wasting/ throwing out" food. I want you to remember, if it's not nourishing you, if it's not helping you move in the direction of your goals, if it's something that could be contributing to creating a lifestyle disease like diabetes, it's not wasteful to throw it away. It's smart, and you're smart. That's why you picked up this book, and you're taking the steps necessary to better yourself and your health. Where do we begin? Let's start with the cupboards or pantry. The dry goods tend to be where most people struggle. Having a kitchen stocked with cookies, pastries, crackers, chips, granola bars, and other snack foods is a recipe for disaster. That's not to say there aren't healthy snack items out there, so we need to distinguish between them.

If something has more than 8 grams of sugar per serving, it should go. If something has a laundry list of ingredients that you can't pronounce, it should go. If something could live in your pantry or on a shelf for years and years and years and not ever actually break down, it should go. You also just shouldn't keep bags of cookies, pastries, crackers, and chips in the house on a regular basis. I get that we like to have snack foods on hand, especially if you have kids. You can have one bag of cookies and one bag of chips; you don't need to have several different types of each. These are foods that should be eaten sparingly by both adults and children, so make that one bag last for at least a week, if not longer, depending on the number of people eating from it.

"I found myself feeling satisfied on less food."

—**Sophie B.**, 26, Independent Team Beachbody Coach, Cincinnati, OH

Sophie B. describes her eating habits as "haphazard, powerless, and naive." She says she had no idea how to properly eat or cook in a healthy way. As a result, she put on pounds and became fatigued, especially after becoming a new mom. With a beautiful 4-month-old daughter, Sophie had every reason to feel joy, but she couldn't smile. She had to fight every day to find the motivation just to get out of bed to tend to her baby girl. "Before beginning the *21 Day Fix*, I was severely depressed and suicidal," she says.

She knew she needed a "guidance course" to learn how to eat healthy and make it sustainable. "My goal was to find out what my body was capable of if I didn't indulge in 'fake foods' and put in it what it actually needed," she says. At first glance, she thought the portion container would never provide enough food. But that changed after 2 days. "I found myself feeling satisfied on less food

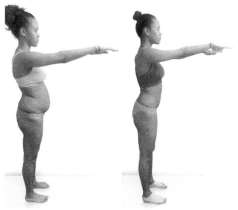

Day 1: 165 lbs.   Day 21*: 150 lbs.

than before because my body was getting satisfied from the food types it actually needed. Crazy talk!"

Sophie lost a total of 15 pounds and 2 sizes following *21 Day Fix* and feels physically and mentally stronger. "I never knew that the bloat and discomfort I was feeling was so related to my daily food," she says. "They always say that abs are made in the kitchen and I definitely found this to be true. I have abs for the first time ever!"

Chapter 3

WHAT'S HOLDING YOU BACK?

You can't start the next chapter in your life if you keep rereading the last one.

As a kid, I was picked on, A LOT, especially by my family. I come from a big Italian family, and that's just sort of how it was. Everyone gave each other crap, but for some reason, I caught the brunt of it from EVERYONE. I was the youngest of my siblings, so I got it from them. I was one of the younger cousins, so I got it from them, and because I was a ball of energy, I must have annoyed the adults, because I got it from them, too. If you ask a member of my family to list some of the "dumb" things I said as a child, any one of them could go off on a tangent, and if there happen to be a few of them around, it would turn into a laughing, make-fun-of-Autumn-fest.

It's bad enough that the kids in the family picked on me, but my uncle did, too. I remember being at Christmas dinner at my aunt's house. Remember, big Italian family, so there are people everywhere. I went running through the kitchen, being chased by one of my cousins, and I bumped into someone who spilled hot coffee on me. I was 7, so of course, I cried. And, as my aunts and grandma started cleaning me and mopping up the coffee, my uncle stood there looking at me in disgust and said, "Autumn, you're such an Autumn."

That's it. That's all he said, but I knew what he meant. He couldn't call me all the names he wanted to call me because adults were around, but the tone of his voice said it all: "You're so stupid."

I loved my family, and to feel that they thought that way about me affected how I felt about myself. They called me Flopsy Mopsy because I was always falling and getting hurt. I felt very dumb and unworthy at a young age. I was always on the defensive, afraid to talk, afraid of accidentally saying something silly or dumb and the ridicule that might follow.

Looking back, I know I wasn't stupid; I just spoke fast. I didn't always think before I asked questions or said things that came out wrong. Sometimes I just made an honest mistake, like saying, "Her dress is green," but she's wearing a blue dress, and you know it's a blue dress, but the words just came out wrong. That feeling of being dumb, of not being good enough, has stuck with me for a very long time. Honestly, it still haunts me at times. But when I found something I was good at, dance, I leaned in hard. I felt I had finally found a place where I belonged, a place where I could shine.

That feeling of not being good enough has defined me. In some ways, it has worked against me. I'm defensive before I need to be. I'm a perfectionist, which happens to work well in my career, but I put a lot of my expectations on others. But, all of the criticism I endured as a child also helped me to become tough and develop the backbone and thick skin I needed for the career ahead of me. Being judged and rejected is an inevitable part of my career. You don't get every audition. You don't land every job. You are critiqued on the way you look and how you present yourself. But my tough upbringing also taught me empathy. It taught me to inspire others, not tear them down. Some trainers yell and use negative reinforcement. That's not me. There's enough of that in the world; I want to be the person who lifts you up in your dark hours and helps you shine even brighter.

Speaking of lifting you up, it's time to get up for a 60-second challenge.

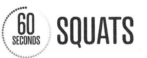 **SQUATS**

A squat is a terrific exercise for building leg strength and a great-looking butt. If you've never squatted before, there are a number of ways to do it:

Easiest: The Wall Sit

- Stand with feet shoulder-width apart about a foot away from a sturdy wall and lean your back flat against it. Now slowly squat by bending your knees until your thighs are parallel with the floor. Try to hold this position for 30 seconds, eventually working up to 60 seconds.

Harder: **Bodyweight Squat**

- Stand with feet shoulder-width apart. Bend your knees to squat. Make sure to push your butt back as if sitting into a chair. Once your thighs reach parallel with the floor, pause a second and then press into your heels and straighten your legs. That's one rep. Do as many as you can in 60 seconds.

Hardest: **Weighted Squat**

- Follow the instructions above but this time hold a 5-pound bag of flour in your hands at your chest to add resistance. You can also hold 2 equal-weight soup cans or dumbbells at your sides as you squat.* Do as many reps as you can in 60 seconds.

* Maintain firm grip and control of weights for safety.

For most people reading this book, *Portion Fix* is not your first time trying to change the way you eat. Maybe you've even tried some crazy diets and didn't lose weight like crazy. It's hard to pick up a book like this, one that's promising you'll lose weight like crazy, and not think back to past experiences, not think back to other times where you've tried and haven't found success, and you will let those other times subconsciously or consciously define your experience with THIS book and THIS method. Instead of letting those past experiences negatively influence your current one, let's flip the script and use them in a positive way. Just like I did with my memories of childhood ridicule. I'm not perfect, so yes, there have been moments throughout my life where those feelings still come up. I've felt I wasn't good enough or smart enough, or worthy, but instead of dwelling on them or even believing them, I flip the script. I used the teasing to fuel me from a C-average student to a straight-A student, not only taking honors classes, but having some of the highest grades in those classes. When I decided to become a personal trainer, I didn't go for the easy certification, I went for the hardest, most in-depth one that I could find. If I was going to learn something, I was going all in. I pay attention, I listen, I learn from those around me, those that have paved the way. I do my own research, and if I don't understand something, I ask questions. Knowing deep down that I am not what other people think of me, I am only what I think of me, has allowed me to move past those limiting beliefs and step into a brighter life than I could ever have imagined.

You can let your past experiences with "dieting" define this experience in a negative way, OR, you can flip the script and let it motivate you.

Here's how you do it:

Flip the Script

Look at past experiences and ask yourself what about it didn't work for you? Was the diet too restrictive? Was it not sustainable for the long term? Did you not understand WHY it worked, the science behind the method? Did you go into it with limiting beliefs that it wouldn't work? Did you give it your all or only half-ass it? What are those past experiences that are defining you, and HOW are they defining you? Think about it, write it down. Now write down how you can flip the script on them, how you can use those past experiences that made you feel LESS THAN to motivate you to be MORE THAN you ever thought possible?

_____

_____

_____

_____

_____

_____

_____

So, what does this all have to do with nutrition and fitness? As I've said before, nutrition is easy: eat your fruit, eat your veggies, pick healthy proteins and fats in moderation, drink your water, don't overeat the junk, and get enough rest. That's the gist of healthy living, so why do we struggle so much? Because we're battling our mind, heart, and emotions, which are very powerful.

Are you eating to soothe that little girl or boy inside of you? Have you healed the wounds that have defined you to this point? That IS a part of nutrition. The traumatic experiences you've endured are there to help build you into the person you are meant to be, but you have to choose how they define you. Do they fill you with self-doubt, self-hate, and self-sabotage or do they build you into a warrior? Do they show you what you are capable of? Do they teach you that the only opinion about YOU that matters is YOURS?

You have nothing to prove to anyone but yourself. So, don't do it for the Holy Shit factor. Don't do it for the F-you factor. Don't do it for the Revenge Body, or I'm-better-than-you. DO IT FOR YOU. Do it 'cause it feels good. Do it 'cause it's good for you. Do it for your health. Do it to set YOURSELF free from the chains that have bound you.

YOU ARE ENOUGH

YOU ARE BRAVE

YOU ARE BEAUTIFUL

YOU ARE WORTHY

YOU ARE SMART

YOU ARE CAPABLE

YOU ARE STRONG

But it doesn't matter if I tell you who you are, just like it doesn't matter if I tell you who you're not. What matters is what YOU believe.

IT'S YOUR TURN
Banish the Negativity Committee

It's time to take those negative feelings you've been carrying around and leave them on the curb to be picked up by the trash. Here's how: I want you to write down every bad thing you have to say about yourself, all those negative thoughts that run through your head on the regular. Go ahead, write them down on a piece of paper.

Read them back to yourself.

Now, imagine that you aren't the one you wrote those things down, that your best friend did, and she handed you that piece of paper. You would feel pretty terrible, right? Would you even think of her as a friend? Well, it's the exact same thing when you think and say those things about yourself. Now, get rid of those negative thoughts. Burn that f'ing paper! Tear it, shred it, flush it. Do whatever you have to do to banish that evil negativity committee in your brain.

Now let's write down what you really are:

I AM _____

I AM _____

I AM _____

I AM _____

I AM _____

"What's crazy is that it took me 20 years to figure this out."

—**Carl Daikele**r, CEO, Beachbody, Los Angeles, CA

Carl Daikeler is co-founder of Beachbody, the man who first hired me to create *21 Day Fix*. You'd think "fitness junkie" would be in his job description as leader of a big fitness/lifestyle company, but not so. Carl doesn't particularly enjoy exercise and his diet is about as nutritious as a 5-year-old's. But that's what makes him ideal as Beachbody's chief: He's just like his customers, the millions of "real people" out there who want to get fitter and healthier but need help achieving their goals.

Like a lot of people entering their 50s, Carl knew he had to make time to take better care of his health, so he embarked on Beachbody's original Power 90 program. "My results with that program's circuit training and sensible eating plan proved to me that if I focused, I could lose weight and get in great shape," he says. "But once the program was done, so were the healthy eating habits."

The pizzas and quesadillas returned and so did his weight. "Five years later

we created P90X, and I did it again; I got ripped and my before and afters were great proof," Carl says. "But I still wasn't eating great. And gradually I slid back."

That setback actually inspired the creation of Shakeology, Beachbody's blockbuster superfood protein supplement shake. "Shakeology gave me more energy and helped me fight off cravings for sweets," says Carl. "I also felt like I was finally getting the nutrition I was missing due to my infantile—but real—fear of vegetables . . . *What's a Brussels sprout? I don't ever want to know*."

Enter *Ultimate Portion Fix* and *21 Day Fix Extreme.*

At age 55, Carl still wasn't feeling as healthy and strong as he wanted to be. So, I challenged him to do the *UPF* program. To my surprise he flipped his priorities, took my advice, and decided to attack the problem first and for the long term by joining my group.

"Before I started the program, I decided

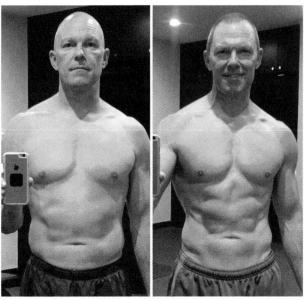

Day 1: **Day 21*: more muscle**

to master the containers," Carl says. "I studied *Ultimate Portion Fix* like I was taking a college class. For a full week I dialed in my nutrition to the letter and finally felt like I had control of what I was eating. Every container was accounted for, and I had a chocolate Shakeology every day." Carl also had the support of my group to keep him accountable. "That's what so many people take for granted," he says. "If I'm not connected to a group doing it with me, I'm left to my own devices, and I know I'm gonna screw up."

But he didn't screw up. Carl lost 5 pounds in his first week. Inspired, he attacked the new *21 Day Fix Extreme Real Time* program. "Intensity is my wheel-house, so once I had the extra energy and confidence that my nutrition was on point and was working online with a group of

other customers who were expecting me to log my workout, nutrition, and shake every day, there was no stopping me."

Week by week, Carl saw the strength and muscle definition of his younger years return. He lost a total of 10 pounds and added lean muscle mass to his body. But here's the big "aha" for Carl: He has maintained that leaner, stronger body for more than a year thanks to having a nutrition foundation and the ongoing support of my *UPF* group.

"Like some crazy breakthrough, I had created a lifestyle that I maintain to this day," says Carl. "After 20 years of running this company, I think that's totally crazy."

So what can we all learn from a crazy busy CEO like Carl Daikeler who used to ignore exercise and eat too much junk?

If he can master portion control in a month and stick with a fitness routine for more than a year, we all can. No problem.

Nice abs, boss man.

Chapter 4

SOMETIMES YOU HAVE TO GO BACK TO GO FORWARD

How I found my passion after losing my confidence.

Are you reliving an emotional trauma from your past?

Is it holding you back? What's the negative story that you keep telling yourself, the painful narrative that's stopping you from letting go and moving forward? Maybe you've tried a bunch of different diets. What about them did or didn't work? Finding these things out can help you go forward with this plan. Maybe you've tried *Ultimate Portion Fix* before, and didn't stick with it. That's OK. You're not starting as a beginner; you've done this before and have that solid base to work from. It's OK to look back in order to see the path forward.

By the time I got to college, I had been dancing for 7 years and competing for 5. I had won multiple trophies, loved the spotlight, and felt confident in my abilities as a dancer. I knew there were many dancers out there who had been dancing WAY longer than me and were definitely better technical dancers than I was. I was OK with that. I just LOVED to dance. Turn the music on, and I feel every beat, every lyric in every ounce of my being. I move, I smile, I perform. I'm in my happy place. That's what dance always was for me. On my good days, I loved going to dance class. On my bad days, I loved it even more. Good day, bad day, dance it out. No matter what was going on in my life, dance class was my place to feel it, enjoy it, or work through it. I still follow that mantra but it has changed just a little. Now I say: good day, bad day, work it out.

As I mentioned earlier, during my junior year of high school, I moved to St. Louis to live with my mom. I continued to dance there. I had great teachers at the 2 dance schools I attended. I even danced for the St. Louis Vipers professional roller hockey team for 2 seasons. For 7 years, I had wonderful teachers full of encouragement who pushed me to be my best and taught me how to fail with pride and get back up.

Then I got to college. I had auditioned and been accepted as a performing arts major with an emphasis in dance. I wanted to do it all—dance, sing, and act. I was living my dream. I went to college knowing nothing other than positive role models in dance. Enter the head of the dance department, let's just call him Bill. To this day I still wonder why he accepted me into his dance program. He knew my background, he watched me audition, he knew what skill level I was at, what my strengths were and where I would need to improve. So why did he seem to HATE me from the minute I set foot on HIS dance floor? Seriously, this isn't an insecurity thing; this man attacked me from the beginning. The more he picked on me, the more stubborn I got. The more annoyed I became in his classes, the less I wanted to be there. Before I knew it, my love for dance was gone. My passion faded into self-doubt, and resentment. At the end of my sophomore year, I needed a break. I took a semester off to participate in the Disney College Program, an internship program operated by The Walt Disney Company. When I returned to school, I was treated even worse. My instructors took my break as a lack of commitment to my craft. I was barely given the time of day except to be made an example of. At one point I marched into Bill's office so frustrated and angry that I didn't care what the consequences of the conversation would be. I basically asked him what his problem was. He told me I had no heart. Anyone ever see the movie *Jerry McGuire*? "No Heart? No Heart?! I'm ALL HEART MOTHER _____ !" I left that meeting enraged, feeling completely defeated. All I could do at this point was put my head down and try to push forward.

I auditioned for the spring show and, shocker, didn't get cast. The department head let me know that he wasn't going to cast me, and because I wouldn't dance in the show, I couldn't graduate. On top of all that emotional trauma, I was in the terrible physical pain I spoke of earlier, with a bulging disc in my lower spine and the near certitude of back surgery if I kept pushing my body the way

I was. So, there it was, I failed. I left college a year short of graduating with a bulging disc in my lower spine, the real possibility of back surgery creeping up, a very bruised ego, and my self-esteem in tatters.

Fast-forward one year: I had been working as much as I could, waiting tables to save every penny. What was I saving for? I was going to Hollywood! That had always been the dream. I would move to Los Angeles and dance at EDGE Performing Arts Center, the school my teacher Gina used to talk about back in Ohio. I was going to dance, act, audition, do what I loved. It was exciting.

When I got to LA, I rented an apartment, started waiting tables, and made lots of actor friends. I took acting classes, got my head shots, and started looking for an agent. But there was one thing I didn't do: I didn't go to the performing arts center to dance. I'd look at the class schedule online. I would even choose one to attend, but I couldn't seem to get in my car and drive to the studio. Every time I thought about going, I heard Bill putting me down, making an example of me in front of the class. "NO HEART."

Taking Baby Steps

The desire to dance again was there, but I honestly believed I couldn't do it, I wasn't good enough. I was in LA for over a year before I finally worked up the nerve to go to EDGE, and when I did, I went to a Jazz 1 class. For some that might not mean anything, but to those who understand dance, this is silly for someone who had been dancing for 10+ years and majored in it.

There was a hip-hop class taking place before my Jazz 1 class started. I was standing outside the room, staring through the window, watching everyone move, sweat, laugh, cheer, and have fun. I was overwhelmed with fear and excitement at the same time. I just wanted that feeling again. The only way to get it was to be brave enough to take the first step. So that's what I did. I slid on my jazz shoes, walked into the classroom, took my spot front and center, and leaned in. The teacher, Jason Young, (now a choreographer for Madonna) was about my age and full of energy and fire. By the time we finished our warm up and across the floor work I was ready to dance. The music came on, and I started to move, before I knew it I was dancing it out. I danced out those negative feelings, and I welcomed in the enjoyment of it all. I continued taking Jason's class for the next several weeks, and at the end of one powerhouse session, Jason called me over and asked, "What are you doing in this class?" My heart dropped. "He thinks I suck, too, I should have never come back," I thought.

But that's not how he saw it. He said I was way above this class's level, and he invited me to his advanced classes at night. That was it, the tiny bit of reassurance that I needed to start building back my confidence. It took 7 years of dancing to get accepted to a college dance program, 3 years of dancing in that program to have my confidence destroyed (let's be honest, it was only a couple of classes before my confidence was gone), 2 years to get the courage to step back on the dance floor and one Beginner Jazz class to start to put the pieces of my passion back together.

Taking that step into Jason's class was my first step toward releasing the limiting beliefs that had been built up from all the years of trauma in college. That step rekindled my love for movement, it brought back my passion. It also gave me the opportunity to meet a friend who ultimately helped me become a personal trainer. That step back reminded me that I wanted to be a person who helped make people feel good about themselves. It was my first step back to my future.

"God bless the broken road that led me straight to you." Any Rascal Flatts fans out there? That song is about the broken road we all walk that leads to our true love. Fitness, nutrition, and helping people—that's my true love. So, yes, God bless the broken road that led me straight to you. Your broken road is leading you, too. So, start again, take it from the beginning, one day at a time, one meal at a time, one pound at a time, one workout at a time, one rep at a time. That's all any of us can do.

Don't Rush the Process, Trust the Process

This is going to be a process. If you've been following a different type of nutrition program, one that limited the hours that you ate or one that eliminated food groups, know that you might have to go back to go forward with THIS program. What do I mean by that? If you haven't been eating carbohydrates for some time, and you reintroduce them, the reaction your body has might feel like a "step back." It's not. What I mean is, there might be a small adjustment period where your body is very happy to have this macronutrient back in rotation, but because it hasn't had it in some time, it might hold on to it for a little bit until it recognizes that there will in fact be a steady supply of carbohydrates coming back in. So, if the scale fluctuates by a few pounds, don't get frustrated. The same goes if you've been restricting the timing of when you eat. I'm going to ask you to eat every 2.5 to 3 hours, all day long. That might be an adjustment for you. There may be times where you're very hungry or times where you're full. Give your body a chance to adjust to this new eating plan. Trust the process.

Don't Fear Fruit

People tell me all the time that they aren't eating fruit because of the sugar. Fruit is not the enemy y'all. Highly processed, sugar-laced food is the bad guy. It's simply not good for you, but fruit does not fall into this category. Fruit is loaded with vitamins, minerals, antioxidants, and phytonutrients that your body thrives on. When you eat fruit in its whole form, you also get plenty of fiber with it. The fiber slows the absorption of sugar into your system, helping you avoid blood sugar spikes. Eating fruit in its whole form can be very good for you. If you've been skipping the fruit, it's time to add it back in. Fruit is delicious and sweet and can be very satisfying when you are having a sweet craving. I like to keep at least 3 different fruits in my house at all times. I eat it after my workout, in between meals as a healthy snack, and I love to add it to my Shakeology to make it even more delicious and creamy. The next time you have a sweet craving, reach for the fruit instead of the cookies. You'll find it to be very satisfying and it will help bring you closer to that goal of losing weight like crazy.

"My core and glutes tightened up. I haven't seen that definition since high school!"

—Ray C., 46, Independent Team Beachbody Coach, Flushing, NY

Pulled rib muscles put a hold on Ray C's fitness journey. He had to take a few months off from working out to recover from his injury, and the pause took its toll. Ray grew up in a restaurant, so he was used to eating huge portions. But without regular exercise, those big meals put on the pounds and he quickly fell out of shape. He became sluggish and tired, and his mental game suffered, too.

"Deep down I always believe I'm capable of so much more than where I am in my life, but I felt hopeless and I lacked drive," Ray says.

Once his ribs mended, he knew he wanted to get back on track healthwise and also pursue developing a business as an independent Team Beachbody Coach. "I wanted to be able to share knowledge of the program to any future customers."

The container system in *Portion Fix* took care of his tendency to eat more than he needed. And the exercise options on Beachbody On Demand quickly helped him burn off the fat he had accumulated over the months of inactivity. "BOD is like having 20-plus trainers at my

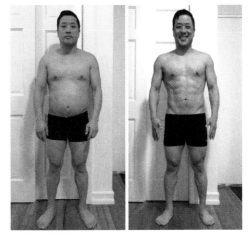

Day 1: 163 lbs.   Day 80*: 152 lbs.

fingertips with over 500 workouts to choose from for the cost of less than one hour if I had hired a trainer," he says. "Can't beat that."

Using my *80 Day Obsession* program and *Portion Fix* containers helped Ray drop 11 pounds and rediscover his energy and passion for life. "I'm carrying less body fat," he says. "I'm stronger and leaner and my posture improved. My core and glutes tightened up. I haven't seen that definition since high school!"

Chapter 5

EVERYTHING YOU EVER WANTED IS ON THE OTHER SIDE OF FEAR

Find the courage, lean in, and push through it.

Repeat this to yourself a few times: Everything I ever wanted is on the other side of fear. Let it sink in.

Now, you might think what's on the other side is the dream job, more money, a big house, vacations galore. While it can mean that, that's not what I mean. What's really on the other side of fear, the thing we all want most, is FREEDOM. When you conquer your fears, you gain a powerful sense of freedom, like you've been unleashed from the shackles that have been holding you back. Powering through your fear makes you realize that you are much stronger—stronger, braver, smarter, and more capable than that thing you feared.

I can't tell you how many times fear has almost stopped me dead in my tracks. When it hits, it hits hard and can be paralyzing. There's a brick in my stomach, a gripping feeling in my throat, my heart races, my anxiety skyrockets, and all of my defenses kick in. Everything in my body screams, "Run, you can't do this, you're gonna fail, you're gonna disappoint people, they'll see you're a fraud and you don't have talent." You've heard of the fight-or-flight response? Well, that's it, but there's no saber-toothed tiger chasing me—the threat is all in my mind.

One situation stands out in particular. I had already put out 3 workout programs with Beachbody and a top-selling cookbook, so I was flying high. Beachbody's CEO, Carl Daikeler, scheduled a meeting with me and told me he knew what he wanted my next 2 workout programs to be. "You like country music, right?" he asked. "Ya, I love it!" I said. "How do you feel about a line-dancing program, of sorts, set to country music?" I told him I thought that could be really fun. "OK," he said, "I'd like that to be your next program. Then we'll talk about creating a butt and abs workout after that."

Carl explained that he wanted the country dance program geared toward beginners. I was excited and went to work. I did my research, learned some line dances, and visited a few country bars to get the vibe and put a routine together for his approval.

But, when I presented what we'd come up with, his response was underwhelmed. "Umm, that's not really what I'm looking for," he said, "I want it to be easy, for beginners."

He was trying to tell me what he wanted, but he couldn't quite explain it past "Easy, for beginners." I could tell he had a vision, but it was up to my team and me to bring it to fruition. We went back to work. We redesigned the program so that, week by week, it progressed from easy to more advanced, then I took it back to Carl. Nope, he still didn't like it. At this point, those demons from my past were starting to creep in: I'm not good enough, I have no heart, no talent, he's going to see that I don't know what I'm doing. I can't do this. My brain was hijacking all reasoning, and I was getting discouraged.

We had another meeting, and this time my fears were confirmed. Carl said we needed the concept and we needed it NOW. We were running out of time to develop the product. I sat in his office with him and the head of product development. He said we were just not getting it, and maybe it was time to switch gears and go with the butt and abs program. We'd circle back to the country program at another time.

That's when the HEART kicked in, and it was stronger than the fear. If I gave up now and switched programs, I knew what would happen: my self-doubt would be affirmed, and it would stay with me forever. Instead, I took a deep breath and said to Carl, "Tell me again, what you're looking for. I just need to get inside your head. I know I can do this if we're speaking the same language."

So, he explained it again: "Simplicity, I don't want people to be frustrated over choreography." Click! Right there, that was it. That was what I needed to hear. I said, "Oh, you don't want dances, you want steps."

"Maybe," he said. "Can you show me?"

I asked him to give me an hour. That's it, just one hour to save my program and reaffirm my confidence. You may think this was the point that I'd feel the most fear, but I knew what was being asked of me, and I knew I could deliver. My heart was my guide, and it could see the future because I wasn't looking over my shoulder for that imaginary tiger.

I grabbed my team, went back into the gym, and put something totally new together. An hour later, I brought my iPad to Carl's office and sat at his desk, nervously watching him watch what I just filmed. Fifteen minutes went by and then he looked up and said, "Yes, that's it. You nailed it. Go create it."

So that's what I did. Was the fear completely gone? Was I ready to move bravely into development? Oh no. We were just getting started. Don't forget I had 3 years of being beaten down by my ballet master, 3 years of being made to feel not good enough, not talented enough. One small victory wasn't going to erase all of that. See, even though you might think I should have all the confidence in the world because of all my other successful programs, this was different. This was dance, the source of all my self-doubt. Developing the country dance program wasn't easy. I was being pushed hard. Cue more, explain what's happening more, make the steps easier. The entire process was challenging me to work through all of my fears, and those frightening thoughts had a hold on me something fierce.

Fear Is an Opportunity to Grow

The universe is always going to test you so you can grow. You have 2 options: buckle under the pressure and live a mediocre life, or rise to the challenge, overcome it, and grow into a better version of you. On any given day, I was rising or buckling depending on the hour. You can expect that to happen to you, too.

We were well into the development of the dance program, and Carl wanted to see where we were at. I was beyond excited to show him. I just knew he would be impressed. At the end of a long rehearsal, I arranged 8 people to show up to dance with me to demonstrate how quickly people picked up what I was teaching. It wasn't just Carl who showed up—the entire development team was there. But I was ready. The music started and we began the routine. I was up there living, having fun, teaching, having one of my rise-to-the-occasion moments. I couldn't see anyone's face while I was teaching because I was so focused on what I was doing. When the 30 minutes was over, I walked up to Carl, smiling, ready for him to praise a job well done. Hahaha, watch out for that first step off your high horse, Autumn, it's a doozy.

Carl looked at me and said, in front of the development team, in an annoyed voice, "That was routine 1?"

I said, "No, that was number 6."

"I didn't ask for routine 6," he said. "I wanted to see 1."
He wasn't happy, and he let me know it in front of the whole team. I
thought it was OK to show him any of the routines, and he thought
he was seeing the very first one, a miscommunication, but he
started to lay into me a little. Not in a mean way, mind you, but
knowing Carl, I could tell he wasn't happy, and I was the reason.
Instantly, the self-doubt took over and laughed in my face, Ha!
And you thought you were rid of me?!

The more Carl talked about what he was hoping to see, the
more embarrassed, frustrated, and disappointed I became. I
was exhausted and emotionally drained from months of battling
my own inner demons. My eyes began to well up with tears. Carl
stopped in his tracks. I looked at him and said, "I'm not being
rude, but we're gonna be done talking now." And I walked away.

I went into another room, so I could cry my emotions out
alone. I was sitting on the floor, tears streaming down my face,
so disappointed with myself, and in walks Carl. He sat down
on the floor in front of me, looked at me, and said, "What's going
on?" He wasn't angry, he knew it was time for compassion. I looked
up and in my shaky voice, still crying, I held up my pointer finger
and thumb barely separated and said, "I'm this close to throwing
myself down an F'ing flight of stairs, just so I don't have to do
this, anymore."

Now, let me tell you that, while Carl is my boss, he's also
my friend. He knows me. He knows when to push and when to back

off. He is an amazing mentor, boss, and coach. So, when I said that, he chuckled a little and gave me a pep talk. He let me know he wasn't disappointed, he fully believed in me, and knew I was capable of putting out an awesome program. He assured me that if he didn't believe in me, he would pull the program, and he had no intention of pulling the program. We talked for a few minutes, and slowly I started to feel better. The inner voices telling me how terrible I was, got quieter. I went back to work, this time with a new belief in myself. Slowly but surely, I worked through my fears, I worked through everything that had been beaten out of me and all the self-doubt that had been instilled in me. The program went on to be called *Country Heat*, and by the time we filmed, it was some of the most fun I've ever had on set. The filming was great, but to this day, if you ask me I will tell you, it's the hardest program I've ever created. That program was there for me to work through all of my B.S., to once and for all let go of the past and step fully into my future.

What was on the other side of my fear? Freedom. I found freedom from what was holding me back, freedom from someone else's opinions and judgments of me. On the other side of my fear, I found a better version of me.

On the other side of fear, you will find a better version of YOU, too. The only way over it is through it, so when it creeps up on you, don't run from it. The lesson will repeat itself until you face it. Lean into the fear and overcome it.

Lean into Fear

Fear can be like a carnival mirror, making small, far-off threats seem bigger and closer than they appear. At the same time, it can make big, beautiful possibilities that are well within reach seem like tiny, impossible objects in the distance. Let's try an exercise to put our fears into perspective:

Write down 4 things about starting this program that make you feel fear:

1. _____
2. _____
3. _____
4. _____

Now, write down 4 realistic consequences if those fears were to prove true.

1. _____
2. _____
3. _____
4. _____

Write down 4 hopes you have while thinking about this program:

1. _____
2. _____
3. _____
4. _____

Now, write down 4 realistic outcomes if those hopes were to prove true.

1. _____
2. _____
3. _____
4. _____

Now compare the first list of consequences to the second list of outcomes. Chances are the first list revolves around stasis, things don't change for the better, but they don't get any worse: I might not lose any weight, the workouts might be too hard for me, I might not be able to give up certain foods. But the second list, that one we based on hope, shows us the possibility of real change: I will get to a healthy weight, I will feel more confident, I will get control of my anxiety. At worst, nothing changes, but at best you accomplish goals you've been waiting years to achieve. I'd say Hope kicks Fear's ass any day of the week.

"The *21 Day Fix* saved my life!"

—**Deon C.**, 30, Beachbody employee, Los Angeles, CA

Deon C. weighed 373 pounds and was almost ready to resort to gastric bypass surgery to solve his weight problem. He began overeating as a kid.

Deon was once tall and skinny. But when his grandfather died, he went into foster care, and that's when the bingeing started. "When you're in the foster system your whole life, you learn to eat when you can because it might not be there tomorrow," says Deon. "I would eat as much as I could even if I was already full, so I didn't have to worry about waiting to go to school the next day to eat again. I never broke that habit: if there's leftover food, I won't put it in the refrigerator, I'll eat it all."

What's worse, Deon says he taught his 10-year-old son the same poor eating habits, telling him, "I don't care if you're full; you will eat it before you walk away from the table."

Today, all that has changed thanks to following the *21 Day Fix* program. "Because of the container system, I can actually put food in the refrigerator to save for another day," Deon says.

Now Deon is teaching good nutrition habits to his son: he no longer overeats but balances his macronutrients to stay satisfied and he has stopped drinking 2-liter bottles of soda at work. As a result, Deon has lost over 111 pounds.

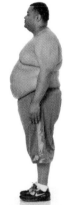 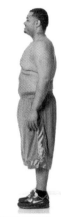

Day 1: 373 lbs.   Day 252*: 262 lbs.

"I was wearing a 6X shirt and size 54 pants; now I'm in 42 pants and a 1X shirt."

"I Was Tricked"

"When first I saw Autumn, I thought, she has no idea what I'm going through. But then I heard her speak, and I listened." After 21 days, he decided to do another round of the program. "I lost another 18, so I was tricked into doing it again and again. The *21 Day Fix* saved my life."

And it has helped strengthen his relationship with his son. "When I was overweight and my son would ask, 'Dad, can we play basketball?' I would always find an excuse because I didn't have the energy," Deon says. "But now, the relationship between me and my son is, like, we're unbreakable; we're best friends."

Chapter 6

THE ANSWERS ARE ALREADY INSIDE YOU

If you are searching for that one person who will change your life, look in the mirror.

Do you ever get the feeling that something needs to change, but you just don't know what it is? You know you can be happier, but you don't know how. You know you could feel better, but you just don't know what you need to do to feel better. What if I told you, the answers are already inside of you?

It was the summer of 2009, just 2 months before my 29th birthday, and I had been living in Los Angeles for 6 years. I began those years waiting tables, then worked as a casting director's assistant before getting certified as a personal trainer and landing a job with a small, in-home fitness company. That's when I began to make a name for myself as a personal trainer in one of the most competitive markets in the world. I was soon able to start my own company and generate a 6-figure income.

I had been married for 2 years and had my son 5 months earlier. Life was going well. I loved my business, loved setting my own hours, helping people, getting to be there for my little family, and most importantly, being the boss of my career and my money. My husband was a restaurant manager, at the time, and had been for many years. He was not enjoying his career like I was enjoying mine. In fact, he was feeling completely burned out. The topic of him switching jobs was one that came up on a regular basis, as was the topic of money in general and how expensive it was to live in LA. I had been encouraging him to apply for a job as a manager at a high-end gym nearby. He's a fantastic manager, but he wanted more normal hours. Going in to work at 4:00 p.m. and not getting home until 2:00 a.m. was getting old. After a lot of discussion, he decided to apply for the management position at the gym.

Good news! He got the interview. Bad news: it was to be a manager at one of their locations in Texas, not LA. "WHOA!" was my only thought at first. I was a little in shock. "Move to Texas?" Did I want to move to Texas? I didn't know how to feel. My type A personality kicked in, and I instantly went into research mode. I started looking for the location of the gym in Texas, began researching the neighborhoods around that area, the rent on apartments, the cost of homes. Then I made my Pros/Cons list. Pros were that my husband could have a job he really enjoyed. I had built my business in LA, so I knew

I could do it again in Texas. My mom lived in Texas, so I would actually be close to family. Cons: Texas is not California. Was I ready to move away from the state I had always wanted to live in? My husband has a son from a previous marriage. Could we really move away? We did a lot of talking. We had a game plan worked out for how we would see my stepson as often as possible. We decided to go to Texas for the interview. While we were there, we stayed with my mom, and she showed us around the town so we could get a feel for where we might live. It was a beautiful town, BUT, it wasn't LA.

My husband went to the interview, and the whole time he was there, I was trying to convince myself that I was excited for him and this would be a good move for our family. I tried to focus on playing in the pool with my son, Dominic. We were splashing around when my husband came walking into the backyard. He had a big smile on his face and said it went really well. He had a good feeling. I told him how proud and excited I was. The next day we got the call. They offered him the job. They wanted him to start in a week! A WEEK! "WTF?"

I went straight into planning mode. As soon as we got back to LA, I started letting clients know I was moving away. These were people I had been training for years; they weren't just clients; they'd become friends. They were sad. I was sad. But I kept in motion, not really ever thinking about the magnitude of what was happening. We packed the apartment and before we knew it, moving day was upon us. I was standing in my empty bedroom with my best friend; my husband was in the living room with our son. I looked at her and tears streamed down my face. She asked me what was wrong.

"This is wrong," I sobbed. "I feel like I'm making a huge mistake. I'm not supposed to live in Texas." She reassured me I was just nervous and it was going to be great. But I knew, I knew I didn't want to go, and yet I felt like I didn't have a choice. We said "yes." We committed. The apartment was packed. It was time to go. We spent the next 2 days driving to Texas.

I tried to stay positive. My husband and I talked about all our plans for our new life in our new town. For a brief moment, I felt like maybe it would be OK. When we got to Texas, we put all of our furniture in storage, since we would be staying with my mom for the first few weeks while we got familiar with our new "home." I hit the ground running, looking for gyms I could work at, making flyers, handing out business cards. Days passed, with no calls from any prospective clients. My husband was at work every day, and he was loving it. I, on the other hand, spent my days taking care of Dominic and crying. I wasn't where I wanted to be, I wasn't where I knew I was supposed to be and I felt it in every ounce of my being.

Now, don't get me wrong. There is nothing wrong with Texas, but my home had become California, and I missed my home. After a few weeks, I got a job as a trainer at a country club. It was OK, but I wanted to be my own boss. I wanted to run my business. I didn't want to work for someone else. On top of struggling to find clients, I wasn't getting along with my mom, which was making living at her house very hard.

Five weeks had passed since we left LA, and I was sitting at the kitchen counter crying to myself again, with no sympathy from anyone around me. I felt trapped, like I couldn't breathe, and I was watching all that my life was supposed to be slip away. For those five weeks, I had tried to convince myself I hadn't made a mistake. I told myself there was nothing I could do; I had made my bed when I agreed to move. I couldn't do what was right for me because I had chosen to do what was right for my husband. So, there I am, crying at the counter, and it hit me what I needed to do. It wasn't going to be easy. It probably wasn't going to go over well. From the outside looking in, I was probably going to look selfish and unsupportive. What did I need? How was I going to be happy? I didn't want to admit what the answer was, but it was there, it was inside me. I just had to be willing to hear it.

My husband got home from work later that day, and I told him we needed to talk. I said to him, "You know I love you, right? I know you need this, and you need to be here, but I NEED to be in LA. I've been gone five weeks now, and if I'm gone any longer, all of my clients will have moved on and everything I worked for will be gone. But, if I go back now, I can still save my business." He began to ask questions about if/when, and I stopped him. I said, "I don't think you understand. I'm not asking you if we can go back. I'm telling you: I'm going back with or without you. You can get a transfer whenever you can, or come with me now, but I'm going back." He understood, in that moment, that this was what I needed to be happy. Two days later, I packed the car up with all of my things and Dominic and I started the drive back to Los Angeles. My husband made the drive with me to make sure we got back OK and then flew back to Texas to go back to work.

That decision to follow my heart, to follow my passion, to listen to the voice inside me saying what I needed, was one of the hardest things I ever had to do, but I'm so thankful that I had the courage to do it. Had I not, I would not be sitting here, writing this book, as one of Beachbody's Super Trainers. I would not be living my dream. The months that followed were challenging, to say the least. My husband was in Texas, and I was in Los Angeles with our 6-month-old. We now had 2 rent payments. I had to hire a nanny to help me with Dominic while I worked, which meant I had to make even more money. But it didn't matter. It didn't matter how hard it was because I was where I was supposed to be. The world felt right again. Just days after I moved back, things started to happen for me. I had reached out to Brooke Burke's team at ModernMom.com and offered to write blog articles for them about pre- and postnatal fitness. They responded immediately and 3 days later called to ask me to go to Brooke's house to film workout videos with her for her YouTube channel. I worked with Brooke for several years at ModernMom.com. Watching her is how I learned to talk to the camera, how I got comfortable with being filmed, so that, several years later, when my opportunity with Beachbody came around, I was ready. You can still find those first YouTube videos of me. They are quite entertaining! I was beyond nervous, and it shows, but it was what helped develop the skills I needed for the career I have today.

The answers are inside you. I knew I didn't belong in Texas, but it took five weeks, a lot of tears, some deep soul searching, and all of the courage to admit it.

Now, let's look at how that relates to helping you lose weight like crazy. Being honest with yourself can lead to hard decisions and breakthroughs. That's what gets crazy results. Personal break-throughs are inside you already, just waiting to be discovered.

The Answers Are Already Inside You

If I asked you what you need to be happy, what would you say?

If I asked you what you need to lose weight, what would you say?

Might these be some of your answers?

- I need to feel worthy.
- I need support to keep me on track.
- I need a plan.
- I need to trust the process.
- I need to stop quitting what I start.
- I need to let go of toxic people in my life.
- I need to leave the job I hate so I'm not so stressed.

- I need to stop eating a bag of potato chips at night.
- I need to stop drinking so much.
- I need to stop late-night snacking.
- I need to exercise more.
- I need to eat more fruits and vegetables.
- I probably should stop drinking so much soda.

You actually already know what you need to do. It's inside of you. So why aren't you doing it? Because it's overwhelming? Because it's scary? Because it seems insurmountable? Because it seems boring? Because you just don't know where or how to start?

OK, you need a little more clarity and a lot more action. Let's start with an exercise to help you gain clarity on what's been stopping you from living your best, healthiest life, and choose ACTIONS to overcome those obstacles.

IT'S YOUR TURN:
Get Clarity and Take Action

Reflect on the following questions. Be honest. Your answers will help you to identify action steps to make positive change happen quickly.

Clarity

What is my definition of health, sound nutrition, and wellness?

_____

_____

_____

_____

_____

Does my current lifestyle help or hinder my nutrition and wellness?

_____

_____

_____

_____

_____

How will improving my nutrition help improve my health and my relationship with food?

_____

_____

_____

_____

_____

What will it feel like if/when I improve my nutrition?

What does a good day of eating look and feel like?

Which limiting beliefs do I still hold that keep me stuck in self-sabotaging behavior?

Do I believe I deserve to be healthy and have a good relationship with food?

Do I look at food as a reward or a punishment?

What would change/improve if I changed the way I look at food?

_____

_____

_____

_____

_____

Action

Do I have a support system to help me improve and maintain a healthier lifestyle? If not, am I willing to meet new people who will help me?

_____

_____

_____

_____

If you would like more support from me specifically as well as a community of people following the same plan, you can sign up for my ongoing nutritional support program The Monthly Fix at TeamACPortionFix.com.

What circumstances or excuses keep me from living a healthy life, including good nutrition and exercise?

_____

_____

_____

_____

How can I surround myself with people who inspire a healthy lifestyle?

_____

_____

_____

_____

What steps am I willing to take to improve my eating habits, and what am I not willing to change?

_____
_____
_____
_____
_____

What new fitness, sports, or activities can I begin as a way of becoming more active and improving my health?

_____
_____
_____
_____

What new mindset do I want to adopt into my life around nutrition and exercise, and why?

_____
_____
_____
_____

How can I set a healthy example for my family?

_____
_____
_____
_____

When I have fun, is it healthy or self-sabotaging? What could I do differently to make my lifestyle and playtime more health-conscious?

_____
_____
_____

With whom or what do I need to set healthier boundaries in order to improve my overall health?

_____

_____

_____

_____

_____

How can I be more knowledgeable about my nutrition and fitness?

_____

_____

_____

_____

_____

Who are my advisers about nutrition and fitness?

_____

_____

_____

_____

_____

What are my most important goals regarding nutrition and health?

_____

_____

_____

_____

_____

Chapter 7

I DON'T BELIEVE IN FAILURES, I BELIEVE IN REDIRECTS

Your next disappointment may actually be leading you to your greatest achievement.

I could tell you I've failed countless times in my life, or I can tell you I've been redirected countless times in my life. As a young adult, I would have used the former verbiage and talked about my failures, but at 39 years old, with a lot of "failures" in my life and the time to reflect back, I can honestly say I've never failed. I've learned, I've grown, and I've been redirected countless times in my life, and they have all been for the better.

Eight years ago, I was a personal trainer working at a very popular, high-end gym in Los Angeles. I had a full client roster, had worked with celebrities, and had been featured in a few publications. I was making a name for myself around Los Angeles. At the time, I had a talent agent who would send me on fitness auditions. I got a call that a popular weight-loss TV show was looking for a new female trainer. I was very excited because this is a show I had watched for years and the thought of having a career like their former female trainer excited me beyond belief. I was so nervous for the audition, but I also knew I could do the job and do it well. I went into it feeling great, ready to show what I could do. The first audition was just an on-camera interview. I went in, did my thing, told my story, talked about the way I like to train people, my method, and the results I'd had with clients. The audition went great, and I got a callback. I was asked to come back a few weeks later. There were more on-camera interviews and some demos of workout moves. I felt really good about the whole process. I was right, and a few weeks later I got another call. This time they wanted me to send in footage of me training.

This was a little trickier. This was 8 years ago, so this was pre-iPhones with their amazing video capability. I needed someone to actually film the footage, and then I needed to upload that to a private YouTube link, where the casting directors could view it. I found a videographer and asked one of my clients if she was willing to let me film her training session, and she happily agreed. I did my thing, uploaded the video, and sent it off. A few weeks later, another call from casting: my audition tapes were making their way up the ranks, but they wanted to see more. This time they wanted to see me training a group of people and, "if they could all be significantly overweight, that would be great, thanks."

Finding several people who had a significant amount of weight to lose, who were available for me to train at the same time, and were all OK with me filming them was much harder. I was determined to land this job, though, so I did the best I could. Again, I went to work. I filmed the training and sent off the new link. A few more weeks went by and another request came in: "Can you do it again and this time can you yell more?"

OK, now I was getting annoyed. I don't yell at people when I train them, that's just not my personality. I'm not motivated by yelling, and I'm not going to try to motivate someone else that way. Remember, I had a lot of negativity growing up; I wanted to be the exact opposite of that. I didn't want to go on national television being anything less than my authentic self, but at the same time, let's be honest, I wanted this job. BAD!

So, one more time I got a few friends together and filmed a training session. I didn't yell, but I did try to bring some tough love to the situation. That was the best I could do and still stay true to me. I sent the link off one more time. At this point almost 3 months of auditioning had gone on. I was definitely feeling good and getting excited about the possibilities. A few weeks after sending that final bit of footage off, I got one more call from the casting director. She said, "It's down to you and one other person. I'm pushing really hard for you. I think you would be great for this.

They are going to make the announcement on Monday. I can't tell you who the other girl is, but if they don't pick you, you'll understand why."

What? What does that even mean? All I could do was wait for Monday. Monday came and I jumped every time my phone rang. I was checking the Internet constantly to see if the network had made any announcements, and then at around 4:00 p.m. there it was online. The new trainer had been announced, and no, it was NOT me. It wasn't even a personal trainer. It was a professional athlete! I was devastated. Four months of auditioning, 4 months of dreaming and getting my hopes up, and they picked another girl. A person who had never trained anyone in her life, who held no certifications, no understanding of what it takes to help someone lose weight in a healthy way? I went home and sobbed on my couch. I remember calling my best friend and saying, "Is it ever going to happen? Am I ever going to get my break? How many times am I going to come this close, only to have another door slammed in my face?" I know what it feels like to want something so bad and fall short of getting it over and over and over again.

My Beachbody Moment

Now, let me fast-forward 2 years: I got the call from Beachbody to go in for a meeting with the CEO. I had spent a year and a half developing a nutrition program called *Change My Plate*, and I had just launched it on a TV show on the Hallmark Channel. I was a one-woman shop, selling the product out of my one-bedroom apartment in Woodland Hills. I would receive the orders, ship the orders, and handle marketing of the product and customer service. I was selling on average 5 to 8 of them a day, which to me was fantastic.

I had given the product to a couple I was training to get their opinion, and they happened to show it to a friend of theirs, who they were trying to encourage to lose some weight. That friend wasn't interested in the product for himself, but he said he knew someone who might be interested and asked if he could pass it along. It's crazy, looking back, how small the world can be. He passed it on to the head of product development at Beachbody. They were very interested, and a few weeks later, I found myself sitting at what seemed like the biggest conference table I had ever seen at Beachbody headquarters in Santa Monica.

I was in a room with Carl, who I mentioned in the last chapter, the company head of product development, and 3 of her staff. Holy crap, Beachbody! Could this really be? Could I actually get to sell my product to the biggest fitness company in the world? I sat there and tried to focus on what the CEO was saying. He asked me how I came up with *Change My Plate* and why I wanted to sell it to his company. He also asked, "If we buy it, would you be interested in staying on as the face of the product and creating workouts to go with it?" UMM, HELL YA, I WOULD!

The meeting was about 30 minutes long and I felt like it went well, but then began the waiting game again. Days went by, then weeks, then 1 month, then 2 months. Just as I was about to give up hope, just as that door seemed to be closing on me again, something amazing happened. At 10:00 p.m. on a Friday night, I opened my email, and there it was, a message from a Beachbody attorney with an offer letter and contract attached! Tears streamed down my face, but this time they were happy tears. I couldn't believe my dreams were finally coming true! I looked at my 3-year-old son, asleep in his bed, and knew in that instant everything I ever worked for was finally happening. Every door that had been closed in my face wasn't actually a door closing, it was more like a train track switching my direction. While I thought I should be going one way to get to my dreams, the universe, God, whatever you believe in, knew better, and was redirecting me to where I truly belonged.

I hadn't failed after all; it just took me a little longer to arrive at my destination than I thought it should. All those times I "failed" were teaching me; they were helping me grow, helping me become the version of me that was ready when this day finally arrived. Looking back now, all I can do is count my blessings that that TV show didn't cast me 2 years earlier. I am exactly where I am supposed to be in my life. I didn't know it at the time, but I would choose to be with Beachbody over that show a million times over. I wouldn't trade any of the bumps and bruises for an easier journey.

When something isn't going the way you think it should, it's almost impossible to see the blessing inside the lesson, but it's there. It might take years to show up, but it's there. There's just one catch: you can't quit. If I had let any of those knockdowns take me out of the game, I would have never ended up here. So, no matter how many times you get knocked down or take a step back, you get back up. And if you're anything like me, you smile and say, "Is that all you got? Bring it on." And you keep on fighting for the life that you want. It's yours if you're willing to do the work and never give up.

It's Your Turn

It's time to start looking at your "failures" as redirects. Can you think of any times in your life that you felt like you failed and reframe them to see the lesson instead? If not, maybe right now is one of those times. Right now, you are taking on something that can be hard—the life change in this program. If you get knocked down, are you going to stay down or are you going to get up and keep on fighting for yourself and your health? Make the commitment right now, to yourself, that you're always going to get back up and push forward.

*CRAZY EASY, CRAZY POWERFUL **TIP #9***

Redirect Your "Fails" with My Help

As you go through the *Lose Weight Like Crazy* program, you might experience some setbacks that you consider failures. Here are 4 potential ways you might "think" you're failing with the program and how I want you to reframe how you look at them:

1. I'm not losing weight as fast as I thought I would.

2. I'm struggling to eat all of my containers, or I accidentally overate on my containers.

3. I do great all week and then backslide on the weekends.

4. I'm struggling with meal prepping; I can't do it.

Here's how to redirect your thought pattern:

1. **Everyone is different and we are all at different places in our fitness journey.** The only person putting a time frame on achieving your goal is you, so remove the time frame. It might take longer than you want it to, but the weight will come off. However, if you quit, that is a guarantee that it won't come off.

2. **This is about progress, not perfection.** Each time you hit a bump in the road, you're being given an opportunity to evaluate what happened around that bump. If you can't eat all of the containers in the day, look at the foods you are choosing. Are you choosing foods that sit heavy? Are there other foods that you can choose that won't be as hard to digest? If you overeat on the containers, ask yourself why? Were you actually hungry? Did you emotionally eat? Did you wait too long to eat? Are you drinking enough water? Maybe you were thirsty, not hungry. Every one of these bumps gives you a chance to look inside and learn more about you and the journey you are on.

3. **Are you setting yourself up for success?** Having a plan for the weekend can make a huge difference to staying on track. Come up with fun things to do that don't revolve around food and alcohol. You might just find some new activities that you really love and even make new friends.

4. **Ditch the word "can't."** Sure, you can meal prep. Don't get overwhelmed by what you see on social media. Meal prepping doesn't have to be some long, arduous process. Stock up on fruits and veggies, pick 1 or 2 simple recipes from this book, and

make those. You don't have to know every single thing you're going to eat for the week. You just have to have foods readily available so that you can grab something healthy when it's time to eat.

AUTUMN'S ATTITUDE ADJUSTMENT

If at First You Don't Succeed...

Congratulations, welcome to life.

It's hard sometimes, but OK. Success doesn't always happen on the first try, and that's OK. Take a baby learning how to walk, for example: if the baby falls on the first try, she doesn't think, "Well, screw it, maybe this isn't for me." In life, it will never be a matter of IF you fall, it will be WHEN you fall, do you accept defeat and quit, OR do you get back up??? We can learn a good lesson from our younger selves, the child inside us that didn't know the meaning of defeat, that wasn't weighed down by society's opinions and all the self-doubt. Things don't always come easy. We fall down, and we rise to try again, and you keep trying because the only time you truly fail is when you quit. Good thing our younger selves never quit, or there would be a lot of crawling adults out there.

(60 SECONDS) MAKE TV TIME CRAZY PRODUCTIVE

25 Crunches
30 Mountain climbers
30 Heel tap hops
5 Burpees

You may be noticing a pattern. Each time I give you a challenge, I'm increasing the number of moves. With baby steps, you are slowly building to a full 30-minute workout!

Part II

YOUR CRAZY PLAN

How to
Kick-start
Your Food
and Fitness
Program

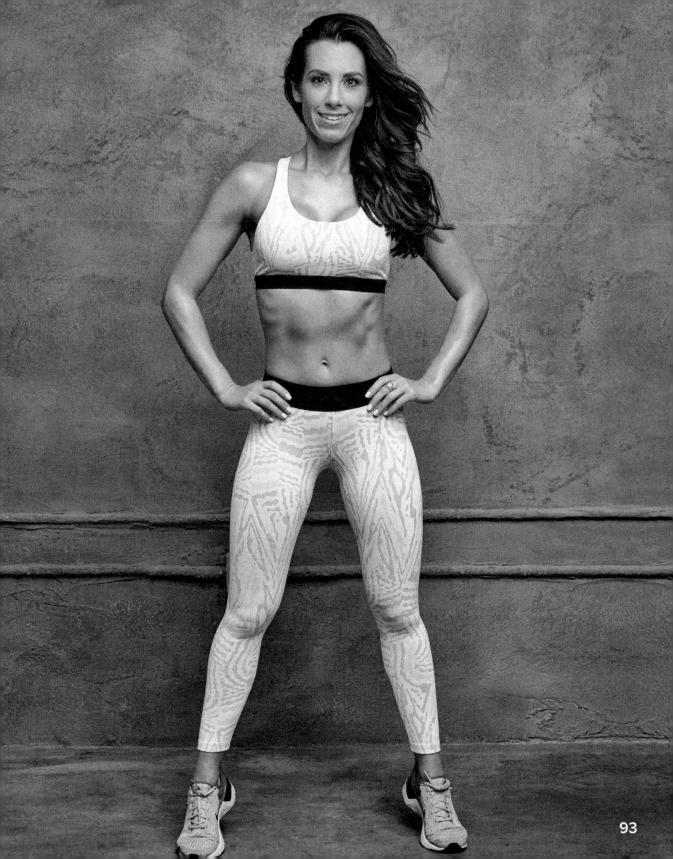

Life Is 10% What Happens to You and 90% How You React to It.

This is the last sentence of my favorite quote. The quote has been my favorite since I was a teenager. I framed it and hung it on my dorm room wall. It stuck with me because of something my dad would always say. Anytime something went wrong he would say, "I'm cursed. It's the Calabrese curse," or in Italian, "What a *malocchio!*" For a long time, that's what I believed: We were just destined for bad luck. Certain people you have in your life, you won't be able to help, such as a father who believes everything bad always happens to him. But be careful of the people you surround yourself with as an adult. Attitude matters, and if you're constantly around people with a negative attitude, chances are, you're going to develop one, too.

Once I was in college on my own, surrounded by like-minded people, having fun and embracing the ups and downs, I started to realize that the manner in which I reacted to situations mattered. I could choose to see the good, or I could choose to see the bad. I could get annoyed, pissed off, or down, or I could learn from my challenges. I started to look at things differently, in a more positive light, and before I knew it, I didn't feel like life was happening to me anymore. I felt in control. The attitude that you bring to this program will determine what you get out of it. If you approach it skeptically, thinking it's one more thing that won't work for you, you're right, it won't. Whether you think you can, or you think you can't, you're right. If you approach it with a positive attitude, asking *What can I learn? How can it work for me?* chances are, you will experience a better understanding of yourself and your nutrition, and you'll get great results.

Check your attitude at the front door. What I mean is, check your attitude at the start of your day. Check it before going into a challenging situation, check it throughout the day. If you go out to dinner with friends and you forgot to save a yellow for your glass of wine, well, you have 2 ways you can look at it: You can be annoyed, think, *this plan sucks, I'm not doing this*, OR you can think, *ah I see what Autumn means about planning ahead and being pre-*

pared. *I'll have water tonight and a cocktail next time we go out. It will still be fun to be with friends.* Having the right attitude will keep you on the path to success.

Attitudes

The longer I live, the more I realize the importance
of choosing the right attitude in life.
Attitude is more important than facts.
It is more important than your past;
more important than your education or your financial situation;
more important than your circumstances, your successes, or your failures;
more important than what other people think or say or do.
It is more important than your appearance, your giftedness, or your skills.
It will make or break a company. It will cause a church to soar or sink.
It will make the difference between a happy home or a miserable home.
You have a choice each day regarding the attitude you will embrace.

Life is like a violin.
You can focus on the broken strings that dangle,
or you can play your life's melody on the one that remains.
You cannot change the years that have passed,
nor can you change the daily tick of the clock.
You cannot change the pace of your march toward your death.
You cannot change the decisions or the reactions of other people.
And you certainly cannot change the inevitable.
Those are strings that dangle!
What you can do is play on the one string that remains — your attitude.
I am convinced that life is 10 percent what happens to me
and 90 percent how I react to it.
The same is true for you.

—Chuck Swindoll

Charles Swindoll is a pastor, author, educator, and radio preacher based in Frisco, Texas.

I share his quote with you because it's a beautiful reminder of how much our attitude matters. Before we dive into how the *Lose Weight Like Crazy* program works, I want you to once again write down what a typical day of eating looks like for you. If you're doing this first thing in the morning, write down EVERYTHING that you ate and drank yesterday. Be honest here, no one else is going to see this. This is for your benefit. We've already done this once, at the opening of the book, but we've also been making a lot of small changes from the onset. Has your eating changed at all since you started reading? If it hasn't that's OK. We're getting into the nitty-gritty now and we will do this exercise again, after the first 2 weeks of following the *Lose Weight Like Crazy* plan, and once more at the 30-day mark, but let's take an honest look at where you are right now.

ONE-DAY FOOD LOG

Breakfast:

_____

_____

_____

_____

Lunch:

_____

_____

_____

_____

Snacks:

_____

_____

_____

_____

Dinner:

_____

_____

_____

_____

Water and other beverages:

_____

_____

_____

SMALL STEPS TO BIG WEIGHT LOSS

It only takes 6 easy steps to lose weight like crazy, even if you have a crazy life. We're going to go over each one in detail, but here they are so you know what to expect.

 Identify your "WHY" and set short- and long-term goals.

 Decide whether or not you are exercising regularly with this plan, and determine your calorie range.

 Find your calorie bracket, and see how many of each container you get to eat a day.

 Make a plan for what meals you are going to eat for the week.

 Grocery shop and meal prep, so you set yourself up for success.

 Track your containers.

That's it; it's that simple. Now let's take a look at each one of these steps, why they are important, and how they work.

STEP 1 Discover and Define Your "Why"

Remember the C.R.A.Z.Y. acronym, from part 1?

Let's start putting it to use. Remember "Y" stands for: Find your WHY for weight loss.

You might have known your "WHY" before you ever even picked this book up, or maybe you discovered it in the first half of the book, as I shared my crazy life stories and how I've overcome some very challenging situations, or maybe your "Why" is yet to fully form itself. That's OK, too, because now's the time to take a deeper look at this important question.

Why is this exercise so important? Wanting to lose weight like crazy is great, and you're obviously motivated right now, while you're reading this. But, what happens in a few weeks when the newness and excitement of this new program and all its possibilities wear off? What happens on that hard day where you think to yourself, "I don't care if I lose weight. Today sucked, and I'm just going to eat this pint of ice cream." I'll tell you. One of 2 things will happen. You'll either eat the ice cream in excess and start down a slippery slope to some old, bad habits, OR you'll lean into your "WHY," your deeper reason for starting this healthy way of eating.

Your "WHY" is what keeps you on track on the hard days. What I've seen, in my more than 15 years in this business, is that wanting to lose 10, 20, or even 100 pounds isn't enough to keep people on track on the hard days. On the hard days, they end up saying, "I don't care." So, you need to figure out WHY you do, actually, care. What are you really working toward?

So, how do we find our deeper "WHY?" Answer these questions:

- What will happen when you lose the weight that you want to lose?

- How will you feel when you lose the weight you want to lose?

- What would happen if you didn't lose this weight?

- How will you feel if you don't lose this weight?

Go deep. Once you've answered these questions, ask yourself, "What else? What else do I need to write down here? What am I holding back from saying, or admitting? Is there anything more that will come from losing this weight?" This will help get you to your "WHY." Once you're there, write it down, think about it, say it to yourself over and over again. I'm doing this to . . .

_____

_____

_____

_____

_____

_____

Setting Goals

Now that we know your "WHY," we can set both long-term and short-term goals. The day you plant the seed is not the day you eat the fruit. I love this saying. A lot of people think losing weight and getting in shape is like flipping a switch—once you decide to do it, you expect it to happen immediately. You eat one salad, and you're standing in the mirror looking to see if you have a 6-pack yet. The day you decide to make a change isn't the day the results of that change will show up. When you plant a seed, it needs a lot of water, sunlight, and TLC. Before you ever see the fruit, you see a little sprout, then a leaf; a bud appears, then blossoms, only to have the petals fall away, and beneath is your first fruit. But it still takes weeks of sun and water and loving care for that fruit to grow to full size and ripen. There are small steps that happen along the

AUTUMN'S ATTITUDE ADJUSTMENT

Repeat This Mantra

I'm doing this . . .

Not for him ➡ but for ME

Not for today ➡ but EVERYDAY

Not to feel good in a dress ➡ but to feel good in my SKIN

Not for the beach ➡ but for my MIND

Not for a competition ➡ but for THE competition I have created FOR MYSELF, BY MYSELF, to become the best version of MYSELF EVERY SINGLE DAY.

way, and some, like the withering of the blossom, may make you feel like you're losing the battle, but they are all necessary on your journey to success.

We know what the end goal is; you probably already have a number in your head as to how much weight you would like to lose. Knowing the end goal is great, but it can also be a bit daunting. So, instead of only focusing on the big goal, we break it down into smaller goals. As I mentioned at the start of this book, achieving each of those smaller goals is what ultimately leads to the big goal. What I always advise my clients to do is determine what the big goal is, then start setting small, short-term goals that will get you to that end result.

A NOTE ABOUT SETTING A GOAL WEIGHT FOR YOURSELF

It's important to have a goal, a direction you are headed in, and often that has to do with the number on the scale. I'm not opposed to this, but I also want to make sure we are clear about determining what that number "should" be. Often clients will say to me, "I'm struggling to lose the last 10 pounds to reach my goal weight." I then ask them how they determined what their goal weight should be: Did a doctor advise a certain number, did they look up their BMI? Nope, the number isn't typically coming from a health care provider. The response is something like, "That's what I weighed in high school," or "That's what I weighed when I was a collegiate athlete," or "That's what I weighed when I was 25, before I had my first baby." Come on, you guys, do I have to point out the obvious?! YOU'RE NOT 17 ANYMORE! When you were in high school you were not a full-grown adult, yet. Your hormones were still changing. Ladies, you were barely at child-bearing age. I'm not saying it's impossible to weigh what you weighed in high school, but it might not be a healthy weight for your body anymore. Same goes for when you were a college athlete. Chances are, you were working out hard most days of the week, maybe playing games on the weekends. Are you hitting the workouts just as hard today? If not, then you probably can't expect to weigh the same as when you were working out that hard. Again, not saying it's impossible, just pointing out what you need to take into consideration before picking a random number for the scale. As you lose weight and, hopefully, build lean muscle from exercise, the most important things to focus on are how you feel, how your clothes fit, and whether or not you are at a healthy weight. This might not be the original number you had in mind, and that's OK.

Let's say the goal is to lose 30 pounds in the next 6 months. Ask yourself, "What do I need to do in this first week to move in that direction?" Week 1 might be, "Reduce added sugars and highly processed foods. OK, I'm going to give up soda this week and clean out my cupboards, so there is no junk food in the house to tempt me." Week 2 could be, "I'm going to start exercising 3 days a-week and meal prep 2 recipes from this book." Week 3 could be, "I'm going to try 3 new vegetables this week." Week 4 could be, "I'm going to add in 2 more days of exercise." See how the small changes feel much more doable and a lot less daunting than, "I'm working to lose 30 pounds." Every week/month, you set new short-term goals that bring you closer to the ultimate goal.

These short-term goals are, "mini wins." Remember, they don't have to be about how much weight you lost this week. Look for mini wins or non-scale victories each week. What's nice about these bite-sized accomplishments is that you can celebrate little victories along the way. If your only goal was 30 pounds in 6 months, you would have to wait until you lost all 30 pounds to celebrate yourself and all of your hard work. It's easy to get discouraged that way because you're not getting that important, regular, positive feedback.

Celebrating Non-Scale Victories

What's a non-scale victory? It's any metric besides the one shown on your scale that helps you evaluate your progress toward your short-term and long-term goals. You'll be surprised how many improvements to your health, physical appearance, emotional well-being, and mood you'll notice as you practice the *Lose Weight Like Crazy* plan.

AUTUMN'S ATTITUDE ADJUSTMENT

Shoot for Progress, Not Perfection

Some quit due to slow progress, never grasping the fact that slow progress IS progress.

Here are some of the benefits you may see while getting healthier:

* Your clothing feels better or fits loser

* You have more energy

* You sleep better at night

* You're stronger in your workouts

* Your skin is clearer

* Your bowel movements are more regular

* You are less bloated/gassy

* You eat dessert without guilt because you practice portion control and substituted it in

* Your body is more flexible

* You have fewer aches and pains

* You wake up feeling refreshed

* You think more clearly

If you are struggling to think of short-term goals, keep this in mind. Successful people set challenging but reasonable objectives, not outrageous ones. Reasonable goals can still be ambitious as hell, but they must be S.M.A.R.T. Maybe you've seen this goal-setting acronym before. If not, here is what it means. S.M.A.R.T. stands for Specific, Measurable, Achievable, Realistic, and Time sensitive.

Specific.

Make sure your goal is not vague in any way; be specific and clear (I will lose 10 pounds in 30 days). And specify your plan: the actions you will take to achieve that goal.

Measurable.

Establish smaller, short-term goals as a way to measure your progress. In the S.M.A.R.T. goal-setting plan, some people use the M to stand for meaningful. I like that idea, too. Goals that are personally meaningful and emotionally connected to you and your set of values are much more powerful motivators. That's why we start with finding your "WHY" before defining your goals. Your "WHY" connects your goals to your heart.

Achievable and Realistic.

Ask yourself: "Is my goal realistically achievable in the time frame that I'm giving myself?" I honestly believe no goal is unrealistic, but the time frame we put on a goal can be. Wanting to lose 100 pounds in a year IS realistic. Wanting to lose 100 pounds in 2 months is NOT realistic. Having a realistic time frame, as well as smaller, short-term goals, is important to reaching the bigger goal.

Time Frame.

We just talked about time frame in setting a realistic/achievable goal. Setting a time frame to achieve your goal adds specificity to it. It adds a sense of urgency and can keep you on track and moving forward. Saying, "I'm going to lose 100 pounds," but never putting a realistic time frame on it can leave you unmotivated to work hard toward your goal.

The S.M.A.R.T. goal-setting template turns dreams into action because it helps you come up with a plan and gives that plan a deadline. The more real and visible you can make your goals, the easier they will be to reach.

It's Your Turn

Set Realistic Long-term and Short-term Goals

- Spend some time sitting quietly and reflecting on your "Why" and what you truly want.

- Write down your main goal. Example: I want to lose 10 pounds in 30 days using the *Lose Weight Like Crazy* plan.

- Now, using the S.M.A.R.T. concept ask yourself, "How can I break down the big goal into small achievable mini goals?"

- Don't forget to include and celebrate the non-scale victories along the way.

- It's not great to focus solely on the scale as a measure of progress. You are more than a number on a scale. You can use it as one form of measurement, but you'll see, later in this section, other forms that we are going to use as well.

- Lastly, if you need help finding deeper meaning in your goals, go back to the Clarity questions in Chapter 6.

THE BASICS OF THE LOSE WEIGHT LIKE CRAZY PLAN

The *Lose Weight Like Crazy* plan is a 30-day kick-start to my *Ultimate Portion Fix* program. I'll be referring to this 30-day kick-start as the *Portion Fix* plan. This program is not something new; it has been around for over 6 years (as of 2020 when this is being written) and has helped hundreds of thousands, if not millions, of people lose weight and keep it off.

To anyone reading this that has already been following *Portion Fix*, or has followed it on and off for the last several years, if you're thinking this is the point in the book where you can stop reading because you already know all there is to know about the program, let me say this: There is a BIG difference between knowing something intellectually and DOING something consistently, to the point where you are living it daily. If you are not living it daily, if it hasn't become second nature (or even if it has), keep reading. Ask yourself: "What else I can learn? How I can improve?" Take it step by step and do the assignments. There is a lot to learn about yourself from the way you look at and use food. Let's dive in.

Practice Consistency

Consistency is what achieves results. Read that again. The key to success, in anything you do, is being consistent. No one makes it to the NFL, MLB, or NBA without practicing consistently, without working to improve just a little bit every single day. The same is true with your health and nutrition. Results take time to get to and forever to maintain. Consistency is what will get you there and keep you there.

As I wrote this book, tragedy struck. On a foggy Sunday morning here in Los Angeles, Kobe Bryant, his daughter, and 7 other people were killed in a helicopter crash in the mountains of Calabasas, just a few miles from my house. I didn't know Kobe Bryant, personally. I'm not a die-hard basketball fan, and yet, since the day of the accident, I haven't been able to stop thinking about who he was as an athlete and the Mamba Mentality. Kobe is a legend, not because he passed too soon but because of his incredible work ethic and talent. I've heard and read story after story about his dedication to his craft from a young age. I've read what his teammates had to say about him, his opponents, his coaches, his family and friends. No one was ever going to out-work Kobe.

For those of you who may not know, one of Kobe's nicknames was The Black Mamba; the Mamba Mentality is defined as a constant quest to be the best version of oneself. No matter how good he was, Kobe always worked to be better, and while I don't know for sure, I have to believe that he never believed he knew it all or couldn't improve. That mentality is something I take with me into all that I do, and I hope you will, too.

WHAT IS THE PORTION FIX PLAN?

Well, let me remind you what it's not. IT'S NOT A DIET!!!
Remember, to me, diets suck. They are the antithesis of the "Z"
in C.R.A.Z.Y. (Zero Deprivation). How many of us have been on a
diet before? You can't see me, but I'm raising my hand. A diet, by
definition, is "a special course of food to which one restricts oneself, to lose weight or for medical reasons." Restricts oneself, yep,
that's the definition of something that's going to suck, in my eyes.
No one wants to be restricted. To be restricted is to not be free,
to be hampered, not able to act at will. No one wants to be restricted,
and once you are, the restriction is all you can think about.
Tell yourself you aren't ever eating chocolate again, and what is
the only thing you can seem to think about? CHOCOLATE.
So yeah, this is NOT a diet.

Portion Fix also isn't about the number on the scale.
What? What the heck, Autumn? I'm reading this book so you can
help me lose weight, and now you're telling me I'm not going to
lose weight?! NO, that's not what I'm telling you. I'm telling you
that *Portion Fix* is about so much more than the number on the
scale. Now, let me tell you what *Portion Fix* is.

Portion Fix is a nutrition program designed to give you food freedom. It is a nutrition program with the specific goal of teaching you how to eat in a healthy, long-term, sustainable way without deprivation or restrictions. When I created *PF*, I wanted to teach people that eating for your health (which will lead to weight loss when done consistently over time) isn't all that hard, it doesn't require starvation, it doesn't require you to give up major food groups, it doesn't require you to isolate yourself from social gatherings, and it doesn't have to taste bad. Check out the 300+ recipes between my 2 cookbooks and cooking show *FIXATE*, and you'll see what I mean. *FIXATE Vol. 1* has sold over 600,000 copies since it launched; if you don't want to take my word for it, you can take all of theirs. With a few basic principles and the help of some color-coded containers, you can completely change your approach to nutrition, and subsequently your health, AND lose weight like crazy. The 3 main principles of the *Portion Fix* plan are Portion Control, Reducing or Eliminating Highly Processed Foods, and Balanced Macronutrients. That's not so hard.

Let's take a closer look at each one of these principles, as well as why they are important. I'm going to go in depth here, but for even more information, remember you can get *The Ultimate Portion Fix* online program on Beachbody On Demand, where I walk you step by step through everything we are talking about here, answer questions that you might have and provide you with all of the tools including a workbook and a logbook to follow *UPF*.

Portion Control

The "C" in C.R.A.Z.Y. stands for control your portions. This is a BIG principle, pun intended. Everything nowadays is supersized, family-sized, and oversized. You are what you eat, AND how much you eat. You don't have to give up foods that you love, but you do need to manage how much of these foods you are eating. Portion control isn't starvation, it's fueling your body for health and wellness. That is our overall goal here. One of the best things about portion control is that it can work for everybody. Vegan, Vegetarian, Paleo, all nutrition theories you can follow with *UPF*, and all can benefit from portion control. Our stomach is approximately the size of our fist. There's only so much food you need to fill it up before you start to stretch it out. The more you stretch out your stomach, the more food you need at the next meal to feel full. Overeating, over time, puts you into a vicious cycle. You overeat, which stretches out your stomach, so you need more food at the next meal to fill your stretched-out stomach and feel full, which means there's a good chance you will overeat again and the cycle continues. This can lead to eating a surplus of calories, which will lead to weight gain. This doesn't just happen with junk food; you can overeat on healthy food, as well. Cue the salad story.

I had been a trainer at a high-end gym, in Los Angeles, for several years, and I had been working with one woman in particular for well over a year. I trained her 4 days a week, and she would also come in at least 2 other days to get a workout in.

This woman was a machine. She busted her ass in her workouts, always giving 100%, and yet, she would lose and gain the same 5 pounds over and over again. I couldn't figure out what the problem was because I knew how hard she was working. When I asked her what she was eating, it all seemed right. Lean protein, veggies, healthy carbs, and fruit. She drank on occasion, but nothing in excess. She was very dedicated. One day after a crazy-hard workout we went out for lunch together. We went to a popular restaurant known for being on the healthier side and both ordered salads. These salads were enormous! While I ate a fraction of mine, she ate her entire salad. It was in that moment that it hit me. I looked at her across the table and said, "That, right there, is our problem."

She asked me what I meant, "It's just a salad." But it wasn't just a salad. It was at least 4 servings of lettuce, 4 servings of chicken, 4 servings of cheese, croutons, pasta, and dressing to cover it all. I looked at the nutrition info on the menu, and sure enough, that salad was over 1,400 calories! That was almost her entire caloric intake for the day, and it was only noon. That's when I started to develop a program based around portion control.

Eating too much at once can also be taxing on your digestive system. The more you put in, the longer and harder it is for your body to break it down and utilize it. Because of this, more of the food you eat ends up stored as fat, instead of being utilized or expelled as waste. Think of your body as a beautiful race car. I love the movie *Fast & Furious*, so let's use the quarter mile as our example here. If you're going to race your car on the quarter mile, does that mean you fill it with fuel until it's pouring out of the tank? No. That's not going to help you win the race, and in fact, it's dangerous to have fuel spilling out of the tank. Same goes for your body. From meal to meal is a quarter mile (you should eat every 2.5 to 3 hours) so you don't need your "fuel tank"/ stomach spilling over with food. You just need to put in enough to get you to the next meal.

By practicing portion control, we are ensuring we are not only not stretching out our stomach, we're not taxing our digestive system, we're staying energized throughout the day, and we're keeping our metabolism revved up. We're also preventing our bodies from storing extra fat because we are only eating enough food for our bodies to use as fuel.

How do we practice portion control? The best way to do this is by using my color-coded portion control containers. You can order them at Beachbody.com. I suggest the containers for a reason. Speaking in color is a lot easier than trying to remember how many ¾-cup servings you get a day. For example, in plan A you get 4 RED containers a day.

RED is your protein container. The RED container is ¾ cup. It's a lot easier to remember "I have 2 reds left for the day" than it is to think "I have 2 more ¾ cups left for the day."

The idea of portion control is not something new. For years people have said, "Eat protein the size of the palm of your hand," "Eat fruit the size of a tennis ball," "Eat fats the size of dice." People have also been advised to weigh their food (eat 4 to 5 ounces of protein), or measure it, (eat at least ¾ cup of protein).

The idea of portion control was there, but it wasn't simplified. My color-coded containers make it beyond easy. Each food group gets a colored container:

■ **GREEN** = Vegetables

■ **PURPLE** = Fruit

■ **RED** = Protein

■ **YELLOW** = Carbohydrates

■ **BLUE** = Healthy fats (cheeses, nuts, avocado, and hummus)

■ **ORANGE** = Seeds and *Fix*-approved salad dressings

●— **tsp** = Oils and nut butters

If you don't want to use the containers, that's OK. I'm giving you the measurements of each container. You'll need measuring cups, if that's the case. The measurements of each container are listed below.

■ **GREEN** = 1 cup

■ **PURPLE** = 1 cup

■ **RED** = ¾ cup

■ **YELLOW** = ½ cup

■ **BLUE** = ¼ cup

■ **ORANGE** = 2 tablespoons

●— **tsp** = teaspoon

As we dive into the program, I will speak about your containers and what goes in them based on their colors. We will take a look at how many containers you get based on the calorie bracket you fall into and the food lists for each container, so you know exactly how to use them to practice portion control. Don't be fooled by these containers. They look small, but once you start filling them and putting the food on your plate, you will quickly see just how much you get to eat in a day.

When you are eating nutrient-dense food, you get to eat more of it. Like I said, you won't starve following this way of eating (Zero deprivation). Before we move on to principle #2, look back at what you ate yesterday. How were your portions? Did you eat a meal that was super-sized or oversized? How did that meal make you feel?

Use smaller plates when plating your food.
We eat with our eyes. When you use a huge dinner plate, putting properly portioned food on it can look small, even though it's a lot of food.

If you use a smaller plate, it looks fuller and will give you the feeling that you are eating a sizable meal.

Reducing Processed Foods

The "R" in C.R.A.Z.Y. stands for "reduce" added sugars and highly processed foods. We need sugar. Our body needs glucose for fuel. The problem is that sugar is EVERYWHERE, and it's being consumed in huge quantities. The problem isn't sugar that occurs naturally in foods like fruit, it's the sugars found in processed, simple, and artificial forms. These types of sugars can lead to all sorts of health issues, including high blood sugar and weight gain.

This is probably the most important principle of the program because, while you can overeat on healthy food, most people aren't doing that. We are overeating on the highly processed foods, the ones loaded with additives, preservatives, food dye, added sugar, salt, and fat. If there is one thing that you can do, right now, to be a better, healthier, leaner, lighter, version of you, it's to cut WAY back on these foods, if not eliminate them completely.

Over the last 70 years, we've turned to fast, processed foods in place of home-cooked meals, and that trend corresponds with the onset of the obesity crisis. We've now reached a point in America where more than 70% of adults and 33% of children are overweight or obese. If you were to ask my opinion about the ONE thing we could do to most effectively reverse this trend, I would say without hesitation, CUT OUT THE PROCESSED FOODS.

The best way to do this is to prepare home-cooked meals

from real, whole ingredients. If you're not used to cooking, fear not. My cookbooks and cooking show have been specifically designed for the novice cook. They focus on efficiency, affordability, and simplicity. You won't spend all day in the kitchen, and if cooking is one of your self-doubts, well, this is the perfect chance to overcome it. If you're not used to cooking, fear not. There are 23 recipes in this book PLUS my cookbooks and cooking show that have been specifically designed for the novice cook.

The problem is, when we choose to eat out, we're not in control of our food. Even if we think we're eating healthy, there is often still a ton of added salt, fat, and sugar, and the portion sizes are far too big. Remember, processed foods have literally been engineered to get you hooked, and restaurants, just like food manufacturers, have a vested interest in getting you hooked on their product.

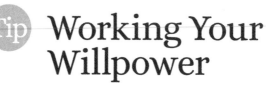

Tip Working Your Willpower

Willpower is an invisible muscle. You have to work it like anything else. Your will is stronger early in the day, but it gets fatigued over time. By the time bedtime rolls around, it's often difficult to resist temptation. Over time, you can build your willpower muscle, but it helps to set yourself up for success by not having junk food in the house to binge on late at night when your will is low.

Balanced Macronutrients

The "A" in C.R.A.Z.Y. stands for "Add" protein, carbs, and
fat in balanced proportions, and that's what the container system
is all about. This principle is a game changer. Even if you're
already eating healthy, there's a good chance your macronutrients
are out of balance. What are macronutrients? Macronutrients are
nutritional compounds that your body needs in significant
quantities for daily functioning. The 3 main macronutrients are
protein, carbohydrates, and healthy fats. Even if you're picking
healthy foods, you might be overeating on carbohydrates but
not eating enough fat or protein. It's important to have a balance
in all 3 of these areas.

Unless you have a specific medical condition, eliminating
one of these macronutrients could be detrimental to your overall
health. We need a variety of vitamins, minerals, and nutrients
to be our healthiest selves. We get these vitamins, minerals, and
other nutrients from all 3 of these groups. You don't need to eliminate a macronutrient group to lose weight. The most popular one
that people tend to reduce or eliminate is carbohydrates. Carbohydrates are not the enemy, ya'll! Highly processed, refined carbohydrates, and sugars are. Overeating carbohydrates can be, but to use
the blanket statement that carbohydrates make you overweight or
unhealthy is just inaccurate. If you're hell-bent on eliminating carbohydrates to lose weight, then this program isn't for you. *The Ultimate Portion Fix* program works with several nutritional theories,

but Keto isn't one of them. To each their own, but I'm with Oprah on this one, "I LOVE BREAD." I also love pizza, fruit, rice, sweet potatoes, wine, and the occasional dessert, so I'm not giving up my carbs, and I'm not going to ask you to, either. But we will have them balanced, and we will have them in the proper portion sizes.

AUTUMN'S ATTITUDE ADJUSTMENT
Eat Like You Love Yourself

Food is not a reward when you do something well. It's not a punishment if you feel like you did something wrong. It's not a coping mechanism to deal with a hard day. Food is fuel. Food is what creates your body. Eat accordingly. Remember, the "Z" in C.R.A.Z.Y. stands for: Zero eating your emotions.

In *Portion Fix* we use a 40-30-30 split. To lose weight like crazy we're going to use a 40-30-30 split of our macronutrients. That means we eat 40% healthy carbohydrates, 30% lean protein and 30% healthy fats. Yes, I put the word "healthy" in front of carbohydrates and fats for a reason. Not every food out there is *Fix*-approved. In fact, not every "food" out there is even really food. Sorry, but if something can live on a shelf longer than I can live life, that's not food. So, we will have healthy carbohydrates, and we will have healthy fats. Double-stuffed cookies might not be approved, but I've got more than one cookie recipe that is mouth-wateringly delicious and won't leave you with a sugar hangover when you eat it.

Why did I choose a 40-30-30 split? *Portion Fix* is not the first program to use this split of nutrients. This is a commonly accepted way of breaking down macronutrients in the nutrition world. The Zone Diet also uses this split, as do many people in the fitness competition arena, which is where I first learned about it and started using it. One of the biggest reasons I like using this split is because your body can only absorb so much of a nutrient at one time. Let's use protein as an example. There's only so much protein your body can utilize at one sitting, so eating an abundance of protein at one meal doesn't mean you'll use it to repair more muscle: it means you'll use what you can and expel or store the rest.

Another reason we use this split is because certain vitamins can only be absorbed when combined with fat or water. Take vitamin A for example; asparagus, kale, and broccoli are high in vitamin A. Vitamin A is a fat-soluble vitamin. In order to absorb it, it needs to be eaten with fat. Sauté your veggies with a teaspoon of olive oil, and you're good to go.

Before we move on, take a minute to think about your meals from yesterday or today. Is there one macronutrient group that you find yourself eating a lot of and another that might be a little shy? Don't worry, we're about to get you balanced out. By using your containers and eating in your proper calorie bracket, you will not only have perfectly portioned meals, you will have perfectly balanced macronutrients. Both are keys to being healthy and both are keys to losing weight like crazy and keeping it off.

Track Your Snack Habits

Quick question: Do you know anyone who binges on fruits and vegetables? Most likely you don't, because natural, whole foods don't send your dopamine skyrocketing the way that highly processed foods and, you guessed it, illegal drugs like cocaine have been shown to do. Artificial sweeteners are hundreds of times sweeter than natural sugars. They provide all the flavor without the actual energy (calories) of the real stuff. Current research shows that this confuses the brain, causing it to potentially crave more sweets later in attempt to get the energy it was denied. It will take time to break the cravings, but as you cut out the highly processed foods, the cravings should start to subside. Tracking your snacking is an eye-opening way to figure out how much added sugars you're eating every day and recognize what may be triggering your cravings. The Snack Tracker below will help illustrate your sugary behaviors. Make yourself additional copies.

SNACK TRACKER

Track your food and feelings, so you can learn more about your cravings.

Date: _____ Wake Time: _____ Sleep Quality: Poor I So-So I Good I Great

Day: S M T W T F S Bedtime: _____

Time of craving	What were you craving?	What you ate	How did you feel after?	What was your last meal before this craving?	Do you have healthy options to satisfy this craving?
				FOOD FOR THOUGHT	
			1 2 3 4 5 6 not hungry starving!		
			1 2 3 4 5 6 not hungry starving!		
			1 2 3 4 5 6 not hungry starving!		
			1 2 3 4 5 6 not hungry starving!		
			1 2 3 4 5 6 not hungry starving!		

SUGAR TRACKER	Breakfast	Snack	Lunch	Snack	Dinner
Grams of added sugar					
Energy and mood after 15 minutes					
Energy and mood after 1.5 hours					

TRACKING YOUR PROGRESS

Tracking your progress is SO IMPORTANT! The scale is just one form of tracking, but it is not the only form, and to be honest, it's my least favorite form of tracking. Why? Because so many things can impact the number on the scale, and end up making you feel like you're not doing a good job, even when you are doing great. If you eat a lot of sodium one day, you might retain a little extra water. Ladies, if you're anywhere near your cycle, the scale will probably go up a few pounds. This again is mostly due to water retention. If you're not having regular bowel movements, that means your body is holding on to waste. Waste has weight. Because of all of these reasons, and so many more, I don't recommend weighing yourself more than once a week, but ideally, you'll weigh yourself on day one of following this program, and again on day 30, and only continue to weigh yourself every 30 days. If you do choose to weigh yourself each week, just know that it's normal for the scale to fluctuate 1 to 2 pounds. You should always weigh yourself first thing in the morning, before eating, and preferably after a bowel movement, if you're someone who is regular. If you're not regular, don't worry. Hopefully that will change with following your new healthy way of eating. I also recommend weighing yourself naked. No need to add extra weight to the scale.

Now let's talk about other ways we are going to track your progress.

WEIGH-IN

The day before you start to follow the plan, weigh yourself and write the number down. Looking at this number, you might feel overwhelmed, you might feel discouraged, you might feel like there's a long road ahead of you. Don't worry, and don't get ahead of yourself. Follow my plan, and this will hopefully be the last time you see that number. That number doesn't define you. It's just a number, let it be just that. It's your starting point, and we're moving forward from here.

PICTURE DAY

After you weigh yourself, it's time for pictures. Grab your phone, put on either a swimsuit or form-fitting workout clothing (you'll want to wear the same thing each time you take your progress pictures). This first photo is your "before" photo. No one else has to see it but you. Having progress pictures when embarking on an effort to change your body can be very motivating. We see ourselves every single day, and that makes it hard to see the small changes, but when you compare your progress pictures each week, side by side, they can show some really great changes.

Stand in front of a clean background—a wall or door is best. If you have someone who can take the pictures for you, that is ideal, but if not, you can take selfies in the mirror, and they will still serve our purpose. Take one photo from the front. Don't suck in, there's no need for that. These are for you, to show you your true progress each week. Next, turn to the side and take a picture, then the other side, and if you can, take a picture from the back—that's great too. You'll want to take progress pictures every 7 days. I typically recommend starting *Portion Fix* on a Monday. That way you can grocery shop and meal prep over the weekend, take your before weight, photos, and measurements, and start fresh on Monday. But, if you're excited to jump in and start, and it's a Wednesday, there's no need to wait, just make sure to do these beginning steps.

BODY MEASUREMENTS

Measurements are the third form of tracking that we are going to use. Measurements can show us the inches coming off, even if the scale isn't moving much. Use a soft, fabric measuring tape to take your measurements. Again, it's ideal to have someone else take your measurements for you, so that they can be as accurate as possible, but if you need to take them yourself, it's not hard at all. Of course, don't measure while wearing bulky clothing. Start at the top, your chest, and work down, recording your measurements on the chart on page 126.

Chest: Measure around the widest part of your chest, over your nipples.

Arms: Measure halfway between your elbow and your shoulder.

Waist: Wrap the tape around your torso over your belly button and be sure the tape measure is parallel with the floor.

Hips: Keeping your feet together, wrap the tape around your hips, right over your hip bones.

Thighs: Wrap around the spot halfway between your knee and hip.

Keep in mind when you're measuring, you don't want to pull the measuring tape too tight. It shouldn't be loose around you, but it also shouldn't be digging into your skin.

TRANSFORMATION TRACKER

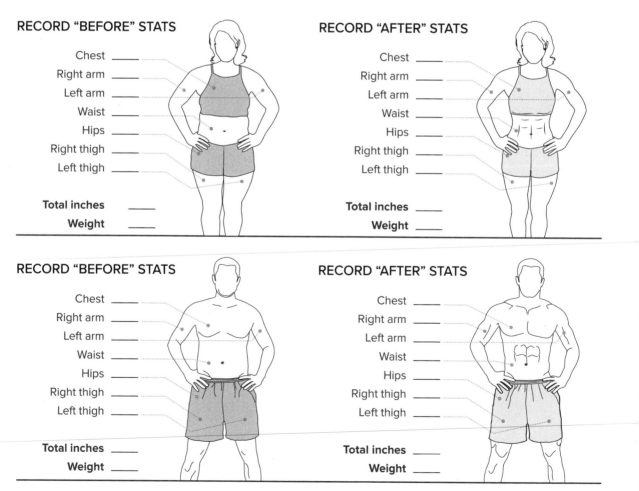

RECORD "BEFORE" STATS

Chest _____
Right arm _____
Left arm _____
Waist _____
Hips _____
Right thigh _____
Left thigh _____

Total inches _____
Weight _____

RECORD "AFTER" STATS

Chest _____
Right arm _____
Left arm _____
Waist _____
Hips _____
Right thigh _____
Left thigh _____

Total inches _____
Weight _____

RECORD "BEFORE" STATS

Chest _____
Right arm _____
Left arm _____
Waist _____
Hips _____
Right thigh _____
Left thigh _____

Total inches _____
Weight _____

RECORD "AFTER" STATS

Chest _____
Right arm _____
Left arm _____
Waist _____
Hips _____
Right thigh _____
Left thigh _____

Total inches _____
Weight _____

CONTROLLING YOUR PORTIONS

It's time to take control of your food, once and for all, instead of food controlling you. I promised at the beginning of this book that eating healthy and losing weight like crazy isn't that hard. Are you ready for me to show you?! LET'S GO!

STEP 2 Decide If You're Exercising or Not

There is no weighing or counting of calories in my plan, but to practice the 3 basic principles, you do need to know how much fuel your body needs. There's a formula for that, and it's the best place to start gaining control of your food. Once you use this simple formula to determine your calorie bracket to lose weight like crazy, you'll know just how many of each of your containers you get to eat a day. No more math after that, until you recalculate 30 days from now.

HOW TO CALCULATE YOUR
CALORIE BRACKET:

First, before you do your calculation, you need to decide if you're going to exercise while following the *Portion Fix* plan. Let me just say this, NUTRITION + FITNESS is the total solution to losing weight like crazy. I even designed 2 different 30-minute workouts—1) Cardio Fix 2.0 and 2) Dirty 30 Sculpt—to get you moving. You'll find these workouts in the back of this book. You can also access them on the Beachbody On Demand app so you can work out with me in the comfort of your home.

If you're not going to exercise, don't worry, you will still lose weight like crazy. Exercising gives added health benefits and allows you to tone and tighten while losing weight, which is why I prefer to combine the two. Once you decide if you're going to exercise regularly, it's time to do your calculation.

This formula is a much simpler version of the Harris Benedict formula, but it gets you to the same place. I wanted to keep this basic to make sure that everyone and anyone who picks up this book can lose weight like crazy. That being said, there are always variables that can come into play. What do I mean by that? Some people are incredibly active, work out for more than an hour a day, have a job that requires a significant amount of manual labor, or might be a breast-feeding momma. For them, there are other formulas that I go into in my *Ultimate Portion Fix* program on Beachbody On Demand. But for the purposes of this book, I wanted to keep it clean and simple, so we will all use 1 of the 2 formulas on pages 130 and 131.

CALCULATE YOUR CALORIE TARGET

To find the right plan for you, you'll need to figure out your Calorie Target using your current weight to find your Caloric Baseline.

IMPORTANT TIPS

- If your Calorie Target is 1,199 or less, round up to 1,200.

- If your Calorie Target is 2,801 or more, round down to 2,800.

- If you want to maintain weight, and are working out,
  stick with your maintenance calories in step 2 of the formula on page 130 and skip step 3.

- If you want to maintain weight, and you are NOT working out,
  stick with your caloric baseline instead of your calorie target.

IMPORTANT NOTE

Your selection of the exercise options is very important.
Overstating or understating your exercise intensity will dramatically affect your results and experience.

IF YOU'RE WORKING OUT

MODERATELY CHALLENGING WORKOUTS 30 to 45 minutes 5x/week: Easy jogging (30 minutes or 3 miles), vigorous hiking, biking (30 minutes)

If your fitness program or daily workout is moderately challenging, you'll use this chart to calculate your Calorie Bracket. Here, we're defining "moderately challenging" as a minimum of 30 to 45 minutes of exercise 5 times a week.

IF YOUR WORKOUTS ARE MODERATELY CHALLENGING

1. Find Your Caloric Baseline
This is how many calories you burn in a day.

_____ x 11 = _____

CURRENT WEIGHT (lbs.)   **CALORIC BASELINE**

2. Find Your Maintenance Calories
Use your Caloric Baseline number to find your Maintenance Calories.

_____ + 400 = _____

CALORIC BASELINE   **MAINTENANCE CALORIES**

3. Find Your Calorie Target for Weight Loss

_____ – 750 = _____

MAINTENANCE CALORIES   **YOUR CALORIE TARGET**

EXAMPLE: Let's use a 160-pound person as an example. The formula would look like this:

160 x 11 = 1,760

1,760 + 400 = 2,160

2,160 – 750 = 1,410

Calorie Target: 1,410

This person would eat in Plan A. You'll see the chart for the different plans on the upcoming pages.

IF YOU'RE NOT WORKING OUT

I recommend you exercise on the *Lose Weight Like Crazy* program. Your results can be better when you do the workouts I've outlined in the back of this book or if you pair this program with a Beachbody fitness program. However, just as with *Ultimate Portion Fix*, you can still get great results by following the C.R.A.Z.Y. nutrition plan without exercising. Use the chart below to find your Caloric Baseline and Calorie Target if you are not working out.

IF YOU'RE NOT WORKING OUT

- **Find Your Caloric Baseline**
  Use this calculation if you're injured or not yet working out other than light walking or stretching.

_____ X 11 = _____
CURRENT WEIGHT (lbs.)   **CALORIC BASELINE**

- **Your Calorie Target**

_____ – 400 = _____
CALORIC BASELINE   **CALORIE TARGET**

EXAMPLE: Let's use a 160-pound person as an example. The formula would look like this: 160 x 11 = 1,760
1,760 – 400 = 1,360
Calorie Target: 1,360

This person would eat in Plan A. You'll see the chart for the different plans on the upcoming pages.

Find Your Calorie Bracket

Once you've calculated your calorie target, find the *Portion Fix* container plan on pages 134 to 137 that corresponds with your calorie target. For example, if your calorie target is 1,300, you'll use Plan A. If you calculate below 1,200 calories, you will still eat in Plan A. You need a certain number of calories a day for your body to function, so we don't want to drop lower than that. If you calculate higher than 2,800 calories, you will round down and eat in Plan F. That will still be a lot of food. The average person needs approximately 2,000 calories a day, so we are staying well within a healthy range of caloric consumption while still losing weight. Find the correct portion plan for you based on your calculated Calorie Target. Your plan is customized for your specific weight-loss needs.

Each plan is color-coded to match the 6 containers, with the number of portions per container listed next to the colored square. For example, if you have a "3" next to the yellow square, that means you'll be filling the Yellow Container 3 times a day. If you are not using the containers, simply portion out the right amount of food based on the guide showing the color equivalents in cups, tablespoons, and teaspoons.

You Can't Out-train a Bad Diet

My plan works, if you follow it, and follow it to a T. For years I've watched people try to out-train their poor nutrition. Guess what? You can't do it, so don't try. Use food for the fuel that it's intended to be, ESPECIALLY if you're exercising. What you eat is what your body is going to become. Do you really want your body to become chips and cookies, after all of that hard work?

Tip

Combine at least 2 to 3 containers at each meal. This will ensure you're getting a balance of your macronutrients at each meal as well as throughout the day.

CALORIE BRACKETS

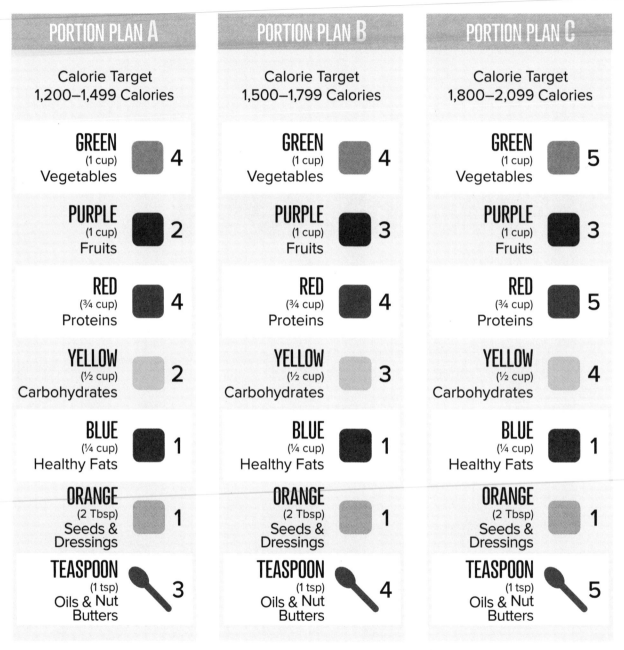

PORTION PLAN A	PORTION PLAN B	PORTION PLAN C
Calorie Target 1,200–1,499 Calories	Calorie Target 1,500–1,799 Calories	Calorie Target 1,800–2,099 Calories
GREEN (1 cup) Vegetables — 4	**GREEN** (1 cup) Vegetables — 4	**GREEN** (1 cup) Vegetables — 5
PURPLE (1 cup) Fruits — 2	**PURPLE** (1 cup) Fruits — 3	**PURPLE** (1 cup) Fruits — 3
RED (¾ cup) Proteins — 4	**RED** (¾ cup) Proteins — 4	**RED** (¾ cup) Proteins — 5
YELLOW (½ cup) Carbohydrates — 2	**YELLOW** (½ cup) Carbohydrates — 3	**YELLOW** (½ cup) Carbohydrates — 4
BLUE (¼ cup) Healthy Fats — 1	**BLUE** (¼ cup) Healthy Fats — 1	**BLUE** (¼ cup) Healthy Fats — 1
ORANGE (2 Tbsp) Seeds & Dressings — 1	**ORANGE** (2 Tbsp) Seeds & Dressings — 1	**ORANGE** (2 Tbsp) Seeds & Dressings — 1
TEASPOON (1 tsp) Oils & Nut Butters — 3	**TEASPOON** (1 tsp) Oils & Nut Butters — 4	**TEASPOON** (1 tsp) Oils & Nut Butters — 5

PORTION PLAN D	PORTION PLAN E	PORTION PLAN F
Calorie Target 2,100–2,299 Calories	Calorie Target 2,300–2,499 Calories	Calorie Target 2,500-2,800 Calories

PORTION PLAN D

Calorie Target
2,100–2,299 Calories

GREEN (1 cup) Vegetables	6
PURPLE (1 cup) Fruits	4
RED (¾ cup) Proteins	6
YELLOW (½ cup) Carbohydrates	4
BLUE (¼ cup) Healthy Fats	1
ORANGE (2 Tbsp) Seeds & Dressings	1
TEASPOON (1 tsp) Oils & Nut Butters	6

PORTION PLAN E

Calorie Target
2,300–2,499 Calories

GREEN (1 cup) Vegetables	7
PURPLE (1 cup) Fruits	5
RED (¾ cup) Proteins	6
YELLOW (½ cup) Carbohydrates	5
BLUE (¼ cup) Healthy Fats	1
ORANGE (2 Tbsp) Seeds & Dressings	1
TEASPOON (1 tsp) Oils & Nut Butters	7

PORTION PLAN F

Calorie Target
2,500-2,800 Calories

GREEN (1 cup) Vegetables	8
PURPLE (1 cup) Fruits	5
RED (¾ cup) Proteins	7
YELLOW (½ cup) Carbohydrates	5
BLUE (¼ cup) Healthy Fats	1
ORANGE (2 Tbsp) Seeds & Dressings	1
TEASPOON (1 tsp) Oils & Nut Butters	8

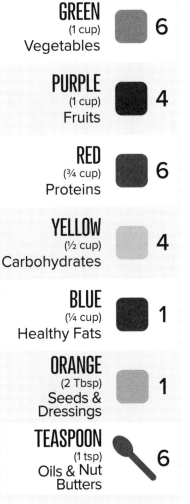
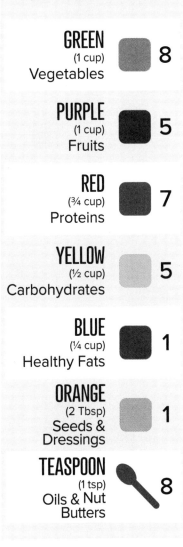

135

VEGAN CALORIE BRACKETS

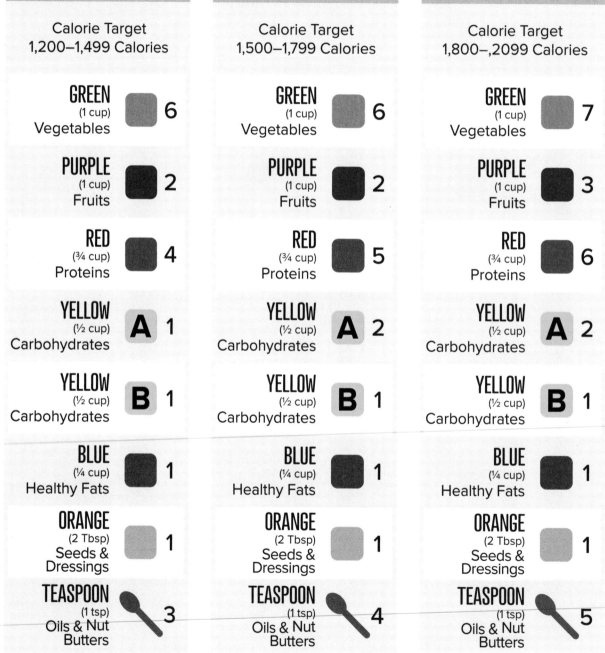

PORTION PLAN A

Calorie Target
1,200–1,499 Calories

GREEN (1 cup) Vegetables	6
PURPLE (1 cup) Fruits	2
RED (¾ cup) Proteins	4
YELLOW (½ cup) Carbohydrates	A 1
YELLOW (½ cup) Carbohydrates	B 1
BLUE (¼ cup) Healthy Fats	1
ORANGE (2 Tbsp) Seeds & Dressings	1
TEASPOON (1 tsp) Oils & Nut Butters	3

PORTION PLAN B

Calorie Target
1,500–1,799 Calories

GREEN (1 cup) Vegetables	6
PURPLE (1 cup) Fruits	2
RED (¾ cup) Proteins	5
YELLOW (½ cup) Carbohydrates	A 2
YELLOW (½ cup) Carbohydrates	B 1
BLUE (¼ cup) Healthy Fats	1
ORANGE (2 Tbsp) Seeds & Dressings	1
TEASPOON (1 tsp) Oils & Nut Butters	4

PORTION PLAN C

Calorie Target
1,800–,2099 Calories

GREEN (1 cup) Vegetables	7
PURPLE (1 cup) Fruits	3
RED (¾ cup) Proteins	6
YELLOW (½ cup) Carbohydrates	A 2
YELLOW (½ cup) Carbohydrates	B 1
BLUE (¼ cup) Healthy Fats	1
ORANGE (2 Tbsp) Seeds & Dressings	1
TEASPOON (1 tsp) Oils & Nut Butters	5

PORTION PLAN D	PORTION PLAN E	PORTION PLAN F
Calorie Target 2,100–2,299 Calories	Calorie Target 2,300–2,499 Calories	Calorie Target 2,500–2,800 Calories

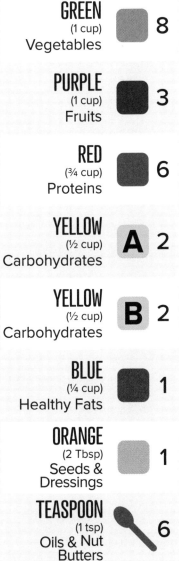

	PLAN D	PLAN E	PLAN F
GREEN (1 cup) Vegetables	8	9	10
PURPLE (1 cup) Fruits	3	3	4
RED (¾ cup) Proteins	6	7	7
YELLOW (½ cup) Carbohydrates **A**	2	2	3
YELLOW (½ cup) Carbohydrates **B**	2	2	2
BLUE (¼ cup) Healthy Fats	1	1	1
ORANGE (2 Tbsp) Seeds & Dressings	1	1	1
TEASPOON (1 tsp) Oils & Nut Butters	6	7	8

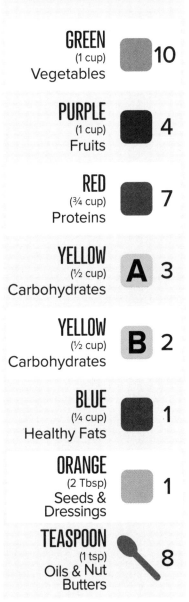

EAT THE RAINBOW

Now let's take a look at what goes in each container. The foods listed are arranged according to their food groups and color-coded containers (if you're using them). Their hierarchy depends on their nutrition value—the higher on the list, the more nutritionally beneficial the food. That doesn't mean you should bypass the foods lower on the lists. A healthy diet supplies a variety of nutrients.

As I mentioned before, my *Portion Fix* plan works for a variety of different nutritional theories—vegan, vegetarian, and paleo being some of the most popular. If you are vegan, you will still use 1 of the 2 calculations from pages 130 and 131, but you have slightly different container counts and food lists.

If you are vegetarian, you have the option to follow either plan, but you need to pick one and stick with it for at least 30 days at a time. If you are a vegetarian who eats eggs and dairy daily, then you will follow the regular *Portion Fix* plan. If you are a vegetarian who eats mostly a plant-based diet and does NOT eat eggs or dairy at least 5 times a week, then you should follow the Vegan plan. When you do eat these foods they will count toward their corresponding container on the regular plan. That means eggs will count toward your RED container as would cottage cheese. Make sure you look at the type of cheese you are eating as some count toward a RED container and some count toward a BLUE container. I go into even more detail on this in the *Ultimate Portion Fix* program, if you would like to dive deeper into it.

NOTE: I've listed many of the foods with specific measurements or amounts for convenience. If you see no amount, just measure out the correct portion with a measuring cup, or fill the container (if using) to the point that you can still close the lid.

VEGETABLES

Green Container

- Kale, cooked or raw
- Watercress, cooked or raw
- Collard greens, cooked or raw
- Spinach, cooked or raw
- Brussels sprouts, chopped or 5 medium*
- Broccoli, chopped
- Asparagus, 10 large spears*
- Beets, 2 medium*
- Shakeology Power Greens Boost, 2 scoops (limit once a day)*†
- Tomatoes, chopped, cherry, or 2 medium*
- Tomatillos, chopped or 3 medium*
- Pumpkin (regular or West Indian), cubed
- Squash (summer), sliced
- Chayote squash, chopped
- Winter squash (all varieties), cubed
- Seaweed (wakame and agar)
- String beans/green beans
- Peppers, sweet, sliced
- Poblano chilies, chopped
- Banana peppers, 3 medium*
- Carrots, sliced or 10 medium baby*
- Cauliflower, chopped
- Artichokes, ½ large*

- Eggplant, ½ medium*
- Okra
- Cactus (nopales), sliced
- Jicama, sliced
- Snow peas
- Cabbage, chopped
- Sauerkraut
- Cucumbers
- Celery
- Lettuce (not iceberg)
- Mushrooms
- Radishes
- Turnips, chopped, or 1 medium*
- Onions, chopped
- Sprouts
- Bamboo shoots
- Salsa (freshly made or pico de gallo)
- Vegetable broth, 2 cups*
- Pickle, chopped

* These food items don't fit in the containers, so just use the indicated amount.

† You can have Shakeology Power Greens Boost as many times as you want each day, but only 2 scoops count toward your containers.

FRUITS

Purple Container

- Raspberries
- Blueberries
- Blackberries
- Strawberries
- Pomegranate, 1 small*
- Pomegranate seeds, ½ cup*
- Guava, 2 medium*
- Starfruit, 2 medium
- Passionfruit, 3 fruits*
- Watermelon, chopped
- Cantaloupe, chopped
- Orange, divided into sections or 1 medium*
- Tangerine, 2 small*
- Apple, sliced, or 1 small
- Apricots, 4 small
- Grapefruit, divided into sections or ½ large
- Cherries
- Grapes
- Kiwifruit, 2 medium*
- Mango, sliced*

- Peach, sliced or 1 large*
- Plum, 2 small*
- Pluot, 2 small*
- Nectarine, sliced or 1 large*
- Pear, sliced, or 1 large*
- Pineapple, diced
- Banana, ½ large*
- Green banana, ½ large*
- Dwarf red banana, 1½ small*
- Breadfruit, ½ small*
- Papaya, chopped
- Figs, 2 small*
- Honeydew melon, chopped
- Pumpkin puree
- Salsa (store-bought)
- Tomato sauce, plain or marinara
- Applesauce (unsweetened)
- Jackfruit (raw in water), ½ cup*

* These food items don't fit in the containers, so just use the indicated amount.

PROTEINS

Red Container

- Sardines (fresh or canned in water), 7 medium*
- Boneless, skinless chicken or turkey breast, cooked, chopped
- Duck breast, cooked, chopped
- Squab, cooked, chopped
- Goat, cooked, chopped
- Lean ground chicken or turkey (>93% lean), cooked
- Fish, freshwater (catfish, tilapia, trout), cooked, flaked
- Fish, cold-water, wild-caught (cod, salmon, halibut, tuna), cooked, flaked
- Game (buffalo, bison, ostrich, venison, rabbit), cooked, chopped
- Game: lean ground (>95% lean), cooked
- Eggs, 2 large*
- Egg whites, 8 large*
- Shakeology, 1 scoop*
- Greek yogurt (plain, 2%)
- Yogurt (plain, 2%)
- Shellfish (shrimp, crab, lobster), cooked
- Clams
- Octopus, cooked, chopped
- Squid, cooked, chopped
- Red meat (extra-lean), cooked, chopped
- Lean ground red meat (>95% lean), chopped

- Organic tempeh
- Organic tofu (firm)
- Pork tenderloin, chopped, cooked
- Tuna (canned light in water), drained
- Lox (smoked salmon), 4 oz.*
- Turkey slices (nitrate- and nitrite-free), 6 slices*
- Ham slices (nitrate- and nitrite-free), 6 slices*
- Ricotta cheese, light
- Cottage cheese, light
- Protein powder (whey, hemp, rice, pea), 1½ scoops (approx. 42 g depending on variety)*
- Veggie burger, 1 medium patty (>16 g protein and <15 g carbohydrates per patty)*
- Turkey bacon (nitrate- and nitrite-free), 4 slices*
- Beef-based broth, 4 cups = ½ ■*
- Chicken-based broth, 4 cups = ½ ■*

* These food items don't fit in the containers, so just use the indicated amount.

Note: Consuming raw or undercooked meats, poultry, seafood, shellfish, or eggs may increase your risk of foodborne illness.

CARBOHYDRATES

Yellow Container

- Sweet potato, chopped or mashed, or ½ small*
- Yams (regular, white, tropical), chopped or mashed, or ½ small*
- Plantains, sliced or ½ medium*
- Quinoa, cooked
- Beans (kidney, black, garbanzo/chickpeas, white, lima, fava, pink, pigeon, etc.), cooked, drained
- Lentils, cooked, drained
- Organic edamame, shelled
- Water chestnuts
- Cassava (yuca), 2 oz.*
- Peas
- Refried beans (nonfat)
- Rice (brown or wild), cooked
- Potato (russet), chopped or mashed, or ½ small
- Potato (red bliss or Yukon gold), mashed or 1 whole
- Parsnips, cooked
- Corn on the cob, 1 ear*
- Amaranth, cooked
- Millet, cooked
- Buckwheat, cooked
- Barley (whole-grain), cooked
- Oatmeal (steel-cut or rolled), cooked

- Muesli/granola, ¼ cup*
- Hominy, cooked
- Popcorn (air-popped), 3 cups*
- Pasta (whole-grain), cooked
- Couscous (whole-wheat), cooked
- Crackers (whole-grain), 8 small*
- Cereal (whole-grain, low-sugar)
- Bread (whole-grain), 1 slice*
- Pita bread (whole-grain), 1 small (4-inch)*
- Waffles (whole-grain), 1 small (4-inch)*
- Pancakes (whole-grain), 1 small (4-inch)*
- English muffin (whole-grain), ½ muffin*
- Bagel (whole-grain), ½ small (3 inch)*
- Tortilla (whole-grain), 1 small (6-inch)*
- Tortilla (corn), 2 small (6-inch)*
- Rice cakes, 2 whole*

* These food items don't fit in the containers, so just use the indicated amount.

HEALTHY FATS

Blue Container

- Avocado, mashed or ¼ medium*
- 12 almonds, whole, raw*
- 8 cashews, whole, raw*
- 14 peanuts, whole, dry roasted*
- 20 pistachios, whole, raw*
- 10 pecan halves, raw*
- 8 walnut halves, raw*
- Hummus
- Coconut milk (canned)
- Feta cheese, crumbled
- Goat cheese, crumbled
- Mozzarella (low-moisture), shredded
- Cheddar, shredded
- Provolone, shredded
- Monterey Jack, shredded
- Parmesan, shredded
- Cotija cheese, crumbled
- Oaxaca cheese, crumbled
- Queso fresco, crumbled

SEEDS & DRESSINGS

Orange Container

- Pumpkin seeds, raw
- Sunflower seeds, raw
- Sesame seeds, raw
- Flaxseed, ground
- Chia seeds
- Hemp seeds
- Pine nuts
- Olives, 10 medium*
- Coconut (unsweetened), shredded
- *FIXATE*-approved salad dressings

* These food items don't fit in the containers, so just use the indicated amount.

OILS & NUT BUTTERS

Teaspoon

- Extra-virgin olive oil
- Extra-virgin coconut oil
- Flaxseed oil
- Walnut oil
- Pumpkin seed oil
- Sesame oil
- Cacao nibs
- Nut butters (peanut, almond, cashew, etc.)

- Seed butters (pumpkin, sunflower, sesame [tahini])
- Butter
- Ghee (clarified butter)
- *FIXATE* Pesto or similar
- *FIXATE* Mayonnaise or similar

Tip

Combine at least 2 to 3 containers at each meal.
This will ensure you're getting a balance of your macronutrients at each meal as well as throughout the day.

Vegan Green Container

- Kale, cooked or raw
- Watercress, cooked or raw
- Collard greens, cooked or raw
- Spinach, cooked or raw
- Bok choy, cooked or raw
- Brussels sprouts, chopped or 5 medium*
- Broccoli, chopped
- Asparagus, 10 large spears*
- Beets, 2 medium*
- Shakeology Power Greens Boost, 2 scoops (limit once a day)*†
- Tomatoes, chopped, cherry, or 2 medium*
- Tomatillos, chopped or 3 medium*
- Pumpkin (regular or West Indian), cubed
- Squash (summer), sliced
- Chayote squash, chopped
- Winter Squash (all varieties), cubed
- Seaweed (wakame and agar)
- String beans/green beans
- Peppers, sweet, sliced
- Poblano chilies, chopped
- Banana peppers, 3 medium*
- Carrots, sliced, or 10 medium baby*
- Cauliflower, chopped
- Artichokes, ½ large

- Eggplant, ½ medium*
- Okra
- Jicama, sliced
- Snow peas
- Cabbage, chopped
- Sauerkraut
- Cucumbers
- Celery
- Lettuce (not iceberg)
- Mushrooms
- Radishes
- Turnips, chopped, or 1 medium*
- Rutabaga, cubed
- Onions, chopped
- Sprouts
- Bamboo shoots
- Salsa (freshly made or pico de gallo)
- Vegetable broth, 2 cups*
- Pickle, chopped

* These food items don't fit in the containers, so just use the indicated amount.

† You can have Shakeology Power Greens Boost as many times as you want each day, but only 2 scoops count toward your containers.

Vegan Purple Container

- Raspberries
- Blueberries
- Blackberries
- Strawberries
- Pomegranate, 1 small*
- Pomegranate seeds, ½ cup*
- Guava, 2 medium*
- Starfruit, 2 medium
- Passionfruit, 3 fruits*
- Watermelon, chopped
- Cantaloupe, chopped
- Orange, divided into sections, or 1 medium*
- Tangerine, 2 small*
- Apple, sliced, or 1 small
- Apricots, 4 small
- Grapefruit, divided into sections, or ½ large
- Cherries
- Grapes
- Kiwifruit, 2 medium*
- Mango, sliced*
- Peach, sliced or 1 large*

- Plum, 2 small
- Pluot, 2 small
- Nectarine, sliced or 1 large*
- Pear, sliced or 1 large*
- Pineapple, diced
- Banana, ½ large*
- Green banana, ½ large*
- Dwarf red banana 1½ small*
- Breadfruit, ½ small*
- Papaya, chopped
- Figs, 2 small*
- Honeydew melon, chopped
- Pumpkin puree
- Salsa (store-bought)
- Tomato sauce, plain or marinara
- Applesauce (unsweetened)
- Jackfruit (raw in water), ½ cup*

* These food items don't fit in the containers, so just use the indicated amount.

PROTEINS

Vegan Red Container

- Vegan Shakeology, 1 scoop* **
- Organic tempeh**
- Organic tofu (firm)**
- Protein powder (hemp, rice, pea), 1½ scoops (approx. 42 g depending on variety)*
- Veggie burger, 1 medium patty (>16 g protein and <15 g carbohydrates per patty)*
- Beans (kidney, black, garbanzo/chickpeas, white, lima, fava, pink, pigeon, etc.), cooked, drained
- Lentils, cooked, drained

- Organic edamame, shelled**
- Peas
- Refried beans (nonfat)
- Seitan

*   These food items don't fit in the containers, so just use the indicated amount.

** Complete protein source with all 9 essential amino acids.

CARBOHYDRATES – WHOLE GRAINS

Vegan Yellow Container A

This is where you'll find whole grains and excellent sources of healthy carbohydrates. Ideally, it's preferable to get most or all of your yellow portions from a Yellow A Container (Carbohydrates–Whole Grains).

- Quinoa, cooked
- Rice (brown or wild), cooked
- Corn on the cob, 1 ear*
- Amaranth, cooked
- Millet, cooked
- Buckwheat, cooked

- Barley (whole-grain), cooked
- Bulgur, cooked
- Oatmeal (steel-cut or rolled), cooked
- Muesli/granola, ¼ cup*
- Hominy, cooked
- Popcorn (air-popped), 3 cups*

* These food items don't fit in the containers, so just use the indicated amount.

CARBOHYDRATES – STARCHES

Vegan Yellow Container B

This container includes tubers and more processed grains, like pastas and breads.

- Sweet potato, chopped or mashed, or ½ small*
- Yams (regular, white, tropical [batata]), chopped or mashed, or ½ small*
- Plantains, sliced, or ½ medium*
- Water chestnuts
- Cassava (yuca), 2 oz.*
- Potato (russet), chopped or mashed, or ½ small*
- Potato (red bliss or Yukon gold), mashed or 1 whole*
- Parsnips, cooked
- Pasta (whole-grain), cooked
- Couscous (whole-wheat), cooked
- Muesli/granola, ¼ cup*

- Crackers (whole-grain), 8 small*
- Cereal (whole-grain, low-sugar)
- Bread (whole-grain), 1 slice*
- Pita bread (whole-grain), 1 small (4-inch)*
- Waffles (whole-grain), 1 small (4-inch)*
- Pancakes (whole-grain), 1 small (4-inch)*
- English muffin (whole-grain), ½ muffin*
- Bagel (whole-grain), ½ small (3-inch)*
- Tortilla (whole-grain), 1 small (6-inch)*
- Tortilla (corn), 2 small (6-inch)*
- Rice cakes, 2 whole*

* These food items don't fit in the containers, so just use the indicated amount.

HEALTHY FATS

Vegan Blue Container

- Avocado, mashed, or ¼ medium*
- 12 almonds, whole, raw*
- 8 cashews, whole, raw*
- 14 peanuts, whole, dry roasted*
- 20 pistachios, whole, raw*
- 10 pecan halves, raw*
- 8 walnut halves, raw*
- Hummus
- Coconut milk (unsweetened)

SEEDS & DRESSINGS

Vegan Orange Container

- Pumpkin seeds, raw
- Sunflower seeds, raw
- Sesame seeds, raw
- Flaxseed, ground
- Chia seeds
- Hemp seeds
- Pine nuts
- Olives, 10 medium*
- Coconut (unsweetened), shredded
- Vegan *Fix/FIXATE*-approved salad dressings

OILS & NUT BUTTERS

Vegan Teaspoon

- Extra-virgin olive oil
- Extra-virgin coconut oil
- Flaxseed oil
- Walnut oil
- Pumpkin seed oil
- Sesame oil
- Cacao nibs
- Nut butters (peanut, almond, cashew, etc.)
- Seed butters (pumpkin, sunflower, sesame [tahini])
- Vegan butter spread or pesto

* These food items don't fit in the containers, so just use the indicated amount.

SEASONINGS & CONDIMENTS

Freebies

Now that you know how many containers a day you get and what goes in them, let's talk about FREEBIES! Who doesn't love something that's FREE?!

- Lemon and lime juice

- Vinegars

- Mustard

- Herbs such as parsley, cilantro (fresh and dry)

- Spices and *Fix*-approved seasoning mixes

- Garlic

- Ginger

- Green onion

- Chili varieties (jalapeño, serrano, ancho, cascabel, pasilla, guajillo, habanero, etc.)

- Hot sauce (Tabasco or Mexican only)

- Anchovy paste

- Cocoa powder (unsweetened)

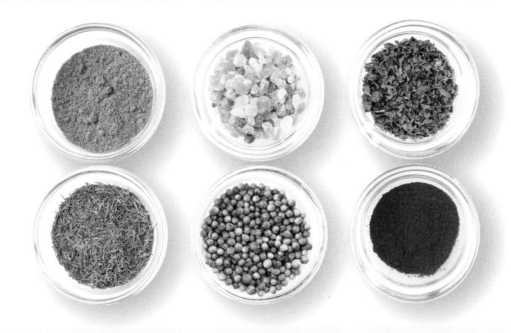

NEXT UP: WATER

Remember my stubborn Italian dad? Trying to get this man to drink water has been a thorn in my side for most of my adult life. For years my dad drove a school bus, so he didn't want to drink water because he didn't want to have to stop to pee. Yes, this was the excuse I would get on a regular basis. On a good day, he might drink 16 to 20 ounces of water. Most days it's a cup of tea here, a small glass of water there, and around 5:00 p.m., out comes the red wine. SMH. I can't even begin to explain my frustration level. He has some pretty big health issues that, in my opinion, could be greatly improved if he improved his diet, starting with his water intake. The body uses water in all of its cells, organs, and tissues to help regulate its temperature and maintain other bodily functions. We lose water not just through sweating, but through everyday life-sustaining activities like breathing, urinating, and digesting, so it's important to make sure we are staying hydrated. Even low levels of dehydration can cause headaches, lethargy, and constipation.

I've heard every excuse in the book for why people don't drink enough water: "I don't like the taste," "I'm not thirsty," "I'm allergic to water." Yes, someone once told me they were allergic to water. If that was the case, they'd have been dead in about 3 days. So, right here and now, let's let go of all the excuses because they are just that. Your body needs water, and there really isn't one good reason that you could give for not drinking it. If you can get your hands on this book, then you can get your hands on some water. Not everyone is privileged enough to be able to say that; let's not take it for granted. If you want to lose weight like crazy, it's time to boss up and drink your water. If you don't like the taste, it could be because of what I mentioned earlier, that you're drinking tap water and tap water can have a bad taste because of everything that could possibly be in it, depending on where you live. So, get yourself a water filter. You can get one that attaches to the sink, or get one that you fill and it filters the water, either way. Filtered water is better for you than tap, anyway. Here are some other ways you can spruce up your water.

The Water Bar

I recommend you drink your body-weight divided by 2, in ounces each day. If you weigh 200 pounds, that's 200 divided by 2 = 100 ounces of water every day to stay properly hydrated. Here's how to make your plain water more interesting:

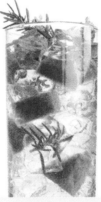
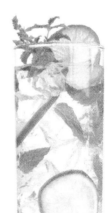
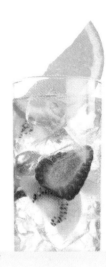

MIXERS   MIX-INS

MIXERS

- Flat water
- Sparkling water (max. 8 fl. oz. a day; make sure it has no calories, sweeteners, or artificial flavors added)

FRUITS/VEGETABLES

- Lemon wedges
- Lime wedges
- Orange slices
- Strawberry slices
- Kiwifruit slices
- Mango slices
- Pineapple slices
- Cucumber slices
- Frozen grapes
- Watermelon cubes
- Honeydew melon cubes
- Blueberries
- Raspberries
- Splash of fruit juice: cranberry, orange, grapefruit

HERBS/SPICES

- Mint leaves
- Basil
- Grated ginger
- Rosemary
- Cinnamon

COFFEE

I can't tell you how many people I've trained that undo all of their hard work by drinking their calories and not even realizing it's a problem. They don't recognize that soda, juice, alcohol, or coffee "beverages" are a huge source of calories. Like most people who love coffee, I love the morning routine of it—the smell when I walk into the coffeehouse, the barista saying good morning and knowing my order, sipping it while driving with the radio up. When I was training clients in their home, and my days started at 4:30 in the morning, I would stop at the coffee shop every single morning and get my usual, a large, vanilla latte with nonfat milk. I never looked at the nutrition info. It was coffee, that's not bad for me. I'd also get a bran muffin to go with it. I really, truly believed I was starting my day off in a healthy way. It wasn't until I started to dive into nutrition that I realized there might be a problem with my morning coffee order. I finally looked up the nutrition information for that cup of joe I was having. Turns out it was a 500-calorie beverage that had 81 carbohydrates in it! Wow! My bran muffin was only 180 calories with 25 grams of carbohydrates in it, but it also had 18 grams of sugar. My "healthy breakfast" was about a third of my caloric intake for the day and more than double the carbohydrates I should have been eating in the entire day! No wonder I was struggling to see results from my workouts, and that was just the beginning. If I had a really busy day I would stop for another latte in the afternoon. Insert palm slap to the forehead here. I'm the personal trainer, and I didn't know any better, that is, until I did.

And once I knew better, I did better. I didn't give up coffee, I just changed my order from a latte to an Americano. I went from all of those pumps of syrup to 1 packet of sugar. I went from the latte, which is basically all milk with a shot of espresso, to my Americano, which is still the shot of espresso but with hot water, and I would add a splash of coconut milk. I took my coffee drink from 500 calories to about 45 calories. I don't want to take away the enjoyment of things like coffee, I just want to teach you better alternatives.

Coffee & Tea

Coffee and tea are fine in moderation. I recommend sticking to 1 to 2 8-ounce cups of coffee or caffeinated tea a day. Herbal teas you can drink all day long. By my definition, "tea" includes regular, decaf, herbal, and unsweetened iced tea. It doesn't include powdered, canned, or bottled tea beverages.

If you'd like to add something to your coffee or tea, here are some ideas and some items to avoid.

Unlimited	In Moderation	Avoid
• Cinnamon	• 1 to 2 Tbsp. low-fat (1% to 2%) milk	• Cream
• Lemon	• 1 to 2 Tbsp. unsweetened nondairy milk alternative (almond, coconut, organic soy, etc.)	• Half-and-half
• Pumpkin spice	• Stevia (1 to 2 liquid drops or ½ single-serve packet)	• Nondairy creamer
• Nutmeg	• 1 to 2 tsp. sugar, honey, or other caloric sweeteners	• Artificial sweeteners
		• Flavored syrups (such as caramel, vanilla, hazelnut, etc.)
		• Chocolate syrup

SHAKEOLOGY

When I started working with Beachbody, I learned about their superfood shake, Shakeology. This took things to a whole new level for me, and I've seen it do the same for countless others. It's a superfood shake with crazy health benefits. It's been shown to help reduce cravings and reduce hunger between meals, and it has superfood adaptogens that can help your body be well. I mentioned earlier that coffee beverages loaded with sugar, syrups, caramel, chocolate, whipped cream and/or sprinkles are NOT coffee! Let's look a little closer. One medium (grande) caramel, blended coffee drink can have close to 500 calories!!!! So, you could drink that, or you could have a RED container of steak, a YELLOW container of mashed potatoes, a GREEN container of sautéed broccoli, and a glass of wine (which would count as another YELLOW) and only be at 370 calories for that meal. I mention that to put into perspective how much food you could eat for the same calories. But, instead of that coffeehouse caramel drink, you could make an Apple Pie Shakeology (see recipe at right). It is amazingly delicious, can be made right at home, and is basically the same price, at just under $5 a serving AND is only 180 calories! Plus, you would get all of the wonderful benefits that come from drinking Shakeology. You can make hundreds of different Shakeology flavors, so it really can be used as a much healthier alternative to just about any coffee-house beverage and more. You can even make it taste like s'mores or cookie dough. These are the choices that people who lose weight like crazy make. That's the bottom line. People who blow off these little extra steps and unconsciously or consciously continue to indulge in those drinks, or who don't find a way to prepare for those sweet tooth cravings, are the ones who continually ask themselves, "Why am I not getting results?" My point is, be mindful of what you are drinking and how that can affect your results. My goal is never to take things away completely, with the exception of maybe soda—that's just a big no-no in my book—but you can have soda water, if you like the bubbles. Instead of telling you not to have something that might be unhealthy, I'm showing you what a healthier alternative is and explaining how it can benefit you on this journey to losing weight like crazy.

Apple Pie Shakeology Recipe

In a blender combine in this order:

- 1 cup unsweetened coconut milk (or milk beverage)
- ¼ cup + 2 Tbsp. unsweetened applesauce
- 1 cup ice
- 1 scoop Vanilla Shakeology (or Vegan Vanilla Shakeology)
- ½ tsp. ground cinnamon

Blend & ENJOY!

Substitutions include treats and other beverages. You may have up to 3 substitutions per week. On the next 2 pages, you'll find Shakeology bases and treats and other beverage substitutions indicating the food group for which you may substitute each.

SMOOTHIE OUT THE "HANGRIES"

When your mood dips with your blood sugar, or you need to crush a craving for sweets fast, blend up a protein smoothie to take the edge off. Beachbody's Vegan Vanilla Shakeology is my go-to fix.

4 oz. water

4 oz. unsweetened coconut milk

1 cup frozen fruit (bananas & strawberries)

1 cup frozen cauliflower (makes it creamy, you don't taste it at all and it gives you a serving of vegetables)

1 scoop Vegan Vanilla Shakeology

- Blend and enjoy.

Shakeology Bases

(ONCE PER DAY)

Shakeology tastes great when blended with just water and ice. It's such a key part of a solid nutritional foundation, I encourage you to drink it every day. But I totally understand if sometimes you want to mix up your routine. Here are some substitutions for water to add variety to your Shakeology experience.

Low-fat milk, 1% to 2% (8 fl. oz.)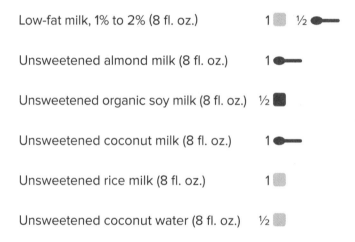

Unsweetened almond milk (8 fl. oz.)

Unsweetened organic soy milk (8 fl. oz.)

Unsweetened coconut milk (8 fl. oz.)

Unsweetened rice milk (8 fl. oz.)

Unsweetened coconut water (8 fl. oz.)

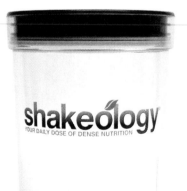

Substitutions

(3 PER WEEK)

Substitutions include treats and other beverages. You may have up to 3 substitutions per week. Below are the foods listed with the food group for which you may substitute it.

Dried apricots, unsweetened (4 pieces)	1 ■
Dried figs, unsweetened (2 pieces)	1 ■
Prunes (2 pieces)	1 ■
Medjool dates (1 piece)	1 ■
Raisins (2 mini-boxes, 3 Tbsp. or approx. 30 pieces)	1 ■
Dried mango, unsweetened (2 pieces)	1 ■
Dried cranberries (2 Tbsp. or approx. 30 pieces	1 ■
Dried apple rings, unsweetened (approx. 7 rings)	1 ■
Dark chocolate, plain (1½" x 1½" square, 1 fun-sized bar, or approx., 25 morsels	1 ■
Potato chips, plain kettle (6 chips)	1 ■
Tortilla chips, plain corn (6 chips)	1 ■

Mini-pretzels (14 pretzels)	1 ■
Peanut butter pretzel nuggets (12 pieces)	1 ■ 2 ●
Chocolate-covered raisins (20 pieces)	½ ■ ½ ■
Chocolate-covered almonds (6 pieces)	½ ■ ½ ■
100% real fruit juice (4 fl. oz.)	1 ■
Wine (5 fl. oz.)	1 ■
Beer, light (12 fl. oz.)	1 ■
Beer, regular (12 fl. oz.)	1½ ■
Hard alcohol (1.5 fl. oz.)	1 ■
Kombucha (12 fl. oz.)	1 ■

You should be drinking mostly water, but I know that can be challenging for some, so here's some beverage guidance to keep you on track.

ALCOHOL

There are 3 beverages that strike a nerve with people when I talk about their health and what they might have to change or cut back on: soda, coffee, and alcohol. Giving up that bottle-of-wine-a-night habit seems to be a deal breaker for a lot of people. This always surprises me. I was doing a podcast interview a few months ago with a very popular reality TV star. We were talking about her getting in shape and feeling her best for her upcoming wedding. I was explaining my *Portion Fix* plan, and she was all-in, right up until I told her she could have wine, but not 3 to 4 glasses a night. She looked at me like I just asked her to give up her first-born child. I reminded her again, "You can have wine, but it's more like 2 to 3 glasses a week, not a night." She just laughed and said, "Oh no, that's not for me." Here is this woman, telling me how important it is to her to feel her best ON HER WEDDING DAY. I say, great here's how we do it, and instantly she decides, nah, it's not that important. So right now, you need to decide just how important it is to you to lose weight like crazy. If your "WHY" is strong enough, this should be a no-brainer. So many people are looking for me or someone like me to tell them how they can continue their unhealthy habits and miraculously lose weight and feel great. They are looking for the magic-pill solution. Honey, there ain't one. If there was, I would be out of a job, and we would all look and feel fabulous living on pizza, wine, and cheesecake. You're going to have to make some sacrifices. You're going to have to change the way you do things. Remember, the "Z" in C.R.A.Z.Y. stands for: Zero excuses.

AUTUMN'S ATTITUDE ADJUSTMENT
Change Nothing and Nothing Changes

You'll only change your life when you change your actions. Change is 100% in your hands, for most people. There is absolutely no reason you can't lose weight, except that you don't want to make the changes that are necessary to do it. If that's the case, that's OK, there's no judgment, that is YOUR CHOICE. But you have to own it. You have to stop saying, "I can't," and start saying, "I choose to look and feel this way," because that is the reality. If you want something you've never had, you're going to have to do something you've never done. Zero excuses.

When I launched my fitness program *80 Day Obsession* in 2018, I dialed up the nutrition component with Timed Nutrition, something you can learn more about in *Ultimate Portion Fix*. With *80 Day Obsession* and Timed Nutrition, I told people there was no drinking for the next 13 weeks of the program. At first, I got all of the typical responses: "You're crazy!" "I can't do that." "I don't want to do that." "That's not possible." So, I hit them with the tough love that I'm now going to hit you with.

If you CAN'T give up alcohol for a few months, then losing weight isn't your biggest problem, and there is someone else that you should be talking to besides me. I don't say that to be mean, I say it to be honest. You shouldn't NEED alcohol to deal with your day or your life. I understand it's a nice way to unwind, it's a fun way to relax with friends. But if it's the ONLY way to unwind or to have fun, then that's an issue that's much bigger than this book.

Besides, with my *Portion Fix* program, I'm not telling you that you have to give up alcohol completely. I'm just saying we have to have it in moderation, and here's how to do it. Oh ya, when *80 Day Obsession* launched, I had over 190,000 people commit to that workout and nutrition program, and the results are mind-blowing. If you want to check them out, just look at #80dayobsession on Instagram. So, giving up alcohol can be done if your goals are big enough and you are determined. Just saying.

"I am 71 years old and I never dreamed I would lose 64 pounds!"

—**Mary C., 71,** Summerville, SC

During a trip to Paris, Mary C.'s son Bradley bought her an outfit and gave it to her when he returned home. "Wow, it's beautiful," I told him, Mary remembers. "I said, 'Let me go try it on.'"

Mary came out with the dress over her arm. "I can't wear this; it doesn't fit," she told her. "He said, 'But Mom, you told me the size.'"

Mary had put on a lot of weight. "I'm more of a yo-yo-dieter, and, um, did it creep up on me," she says. Mary felt terrible. She told her son, 'I'm sorry, but I will get into that dress someday."

For some time, she didn't feel comfortable in her clothing. She didn't enjoy attending gatherings and parties because of her weight. She used to suck in her stomach when she was around people. She was determined to slim down, so she began the *21 Day Fix*.

Each week, she lost weight—2 pounds, then 4 pounds. One week she lost 10 pounds. "I was ecstatic."

Controlling portions and eating the

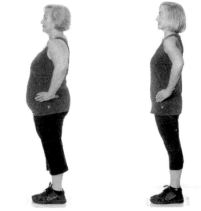

Day 1: 198 lbs.   Day 210*: 134 lbs.

right ratio of proteins, fats, and carbs erased years of consuming unhealthy foods. And she found the exercises "not hard at all; easy for a 71-year-old woman to do," she says.

After 7 months on my program, Mary lost 64 pounds and many inches from her waist. "I'm rockin' out my skinny jeans now," says Mary. And today she can slip into that outfit that Bradley bought her in Paris. "It's larger than me; I will have to have alterations done," Mary says. "It's just phenomenal."

Being Prepared Isn't Half the Battle, It Is the Battle

In order to lose weight like crazy, you're going to need to be prepared. I don't mean mentally, although that is important, too. I mean you actually need to take action steps to be successful with this plan. Following the plan is quite easy, IF you are prepared.

The first step is preparing your kitchen for success. You don't need a bunch of fancy appliances and utensils to cook healthy meals, but having a few basic things on hand will help you make delicious meals, especially *FIXATE* meals, for yourself and your family. Below is a list of things that are good to have in your kitchen. If you don't have all of them, that's OK, you can add things in over time.

Kitchen Gadgets:

- Blender (good for making Shakeology, but also lots of *FIXATE* recipes)
- Set of pots and pans (at least one medium frying pan and one medium soup pan to get you going)
- Rubber spatula, slotted wooden spoon
- Measuring cups and spoons
- Cheese grater/zester

Storage Containers:

- *Portion Fix* color-coded containers. These are ideal for following my *Portion Fix* plan. They are microwave- and top-shelf-dishwasher-safe, plus travel well for meals on the go.

- Ziplock baggies, small and medium

- Glass salad dressing bottle and/or mason jars. These are good for storing *FIXATE* soups, salad dressings, and sauces.

- Plastic wrap, parchment paper, and aluminum foil for covering foods.

Pantry:

- Brown or wild rice
- Oats, steel-cut or rolled
- Quinoa
- Canned beans
- Gluten-free all-purpose flour
- Baking powder
- Baking soda
- Sea salt
- Variety of spices and seasonings (black pepper, garlic powder, onion powder, cumin, rosemary, thyme, cinnamon, nutmeg)
- Honey
- Pure maple syrup
- Olive oil
- Coconut oil
- Vinegar (balsamic, red, or white)

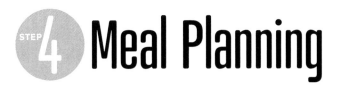 **Meal Planning**

Let's talk Meal Planning: Each week before you go to the grocery store, it's important to plan at least some of the meals you are going to make for the week. Remember, being prepared isn't half the battle, it is the battle. It's time to win this one. I often hear that eating healthy is expensive. Well, it doesn't have to be if you plan for it and stick to that plan. Below is my easy, 3-step process that keeps it simple for meal planning. If you are brand-new to this way of eating, I suggest you keep things very simple. You can start by combining foods from the food lists to make a meal. I suggest combining at least 3 containers to make a meal and at least 2 for a snack. A great meal combination is a RED, YELLOW, GREEN, tsp. As for a snack, I like putting a BLUE and a GREEN together or a PURPLE and a tsp. If you are feeling adventurous, you can pick 1 to 2 recipes from the back of this book to prepare for the week. If you are an avid "chef," someone who loves to cook, then you might want to check out one of my cookbooks, *FIXATE Vol. 1* or *FIXATE Vol. 2*, as well as my cooking show, *FIXATE* on Beachbody On Demand. You'll find hundreds of recipes, including breakfast, lunch, dinner, desserts, snacks, side dishes, holiday recipes, and cocktails—all approved to help you lose weight like crazy and all crazy delicious. But for now, let's keep it simple.

1. Think about what types of food you would like to make for breakfast, lunch, and dinner this week. Keeping in mind, it's OK to have the same thing more than once, to be efficient. That means you can have eggs or oatmeal for breakfast more than once this week. If you buy chicken breast and grill it, you can have it for dinner one night and lunch the next day.

2. Take stock in what you already have on hand and what you need. Then, make a list of which ingredients you will need from the grocery store for the week.

3. Hit the grocery store to get the items on your list. ONLY BUY

WHAT IS ON YOUR LIST. It's ideal to not go to the grocery store hungry. When you do, you typically end up buying more food and more foods that you shouldn't eat. Make sure that you are well stocked on foods for each of your color-coded containers.

If you would like more tools for meal planning, you can check out *Ultimate Portion Fix* on Beachbody On Demand. There, I provide downloadable PDFs that you can fill in for your grocery list, as well as your meal plans. I also provide one-day sample meal plans for every calorie bracket (both regular and vegan plan). This can help give you an idea of how to combine your containers as well as easy meals that you can start with.

GROCERY SHOPPING TIPS:

I always keep my refrigerator stocked with frozen fruits and veggies. Frozen fruit is great to throw in a shake or even to sauté up with a drizzle of maple syrup, cinnamon, and vanilla extract for a healthy "dessert." Frozen veggies come in handy if something is out of season or if you are running low on fresh veggies for the week. A lot of times frozen fruit and vegetables have a higher nutritional value than fresh. That's because they are picked at the peak of freshness and flash-frozen on the spot, so they retain more of their nutrients. Depending on where you buy your fresh produce, it might have traveled on a truck for several days before hitting the supermarket shelf, then it sits on the shelf for at least a few days, so by the time you eat it, it might already be 2 weeks old.

When you first start the *Portion Fix* program it will take a little getting used to to know exactly how much produce you need to buy.

If you find that you've bought too much fruit and veggies and you're not going to get to use them all before they go bad, chop them up and put them in the freezer to use later in soups, stews, and smoothies.

If you live in an area that has local farmer's markets, I suggest shopping there. Usually the farmers are coming from within a 30- to 40-mile radius, so your food is locally grown. It's typically picked a day or 2 before bringing it to market, so it's fresh, and it's a great way to support your local farmers. A lot of times this is a great way to get produce that is technically grown organic but might not have the label, at a more affordable price. It's expensive to become "certified organic." A lot of smaller farms can't afford the certification, but they still abide by the practices of being organic. So, you can often find better prices for "organic" produce at farmer's markets.

If you're going to buy fruit or vegetables that have been canned, be aware that sodium and preservatives could have been added. Read your labels. Make sure it says, "no sodium added," and make sure your fruit is in its own natural juice, not in syrup. That is just extra, unnecessary sugar.

When you're grocery shopping, you're going to want to avoid buying food products with certain catchy phrases on them or certain ingredients—phrases like "low-calorie," "reduced calorie," and "zero calorie," to name a few. This can lead you to believe you are buying something that is healthier for you than its counterpart, with all its fat or natural sugars, but when sugar and/or fat have been removed, usually something else has been added in to make it taste good, and that something else usually is fake and not so great for your body. If something is truly natural and good for you, it doesn't typically need a lot of food labeling to tell you that. I mean, I've never seen broccoli labeled reduced sugar or an apple labeled low-fat. Just saying.

When it comes to sugar, this can be a sneaky ingredient. There are over 60 different names for sugar that can be used on food packages. Hidden sugars can wreak havoc on your weight and your health. Some common names for sugar are

- Dextrose
- Evaporated Cane Juice
- Fructose
- Galactose
- Glucose
- High-Fructose Corn Syrup
- Lactose
- Maltose
- Sucrose
- Tapioca Syrup

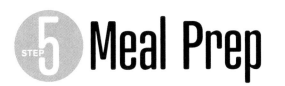 # Meal Prep

Once you've meal planned, it's time to meal prep. This can feel very overwhelming to a lot of people. If you go on social media, you see all these beautiful pictures of people's perfectly organized fridges, filled with containers of their meal prepped food, and you probably think to yourself, "I don't have time for that." Yeah, me neither. Again, I'm going to encourage you to keep it simple, for now. I prefer to meal prep in bulk. That means, instead of preparing all of my meals for the entire week, I cook a few things in bulk and mix and match items throughout the week. I might cook turkey taco meat and grilled chicken breast, and then keep ground beef in the fridge to make burgers later in the week. I'll also cook off a batch of brown rice and bake a sweet potato or 2, since these things take longer to cook. Other than that, I keep fresh vegetables on hand that I can eat raw, or cook and add to my protein and carbohydrates. I also keep 2 to 3 different types of fresh fruit on hand that I can grab as a snack. I'll usually keep avocados or guacamole stocked for my BLUE container, and I make at least one *FIXATE* salad dressing a week that I can use on a salad, to dip veggies in, or as a marinade for my protein, and that counts as an ORANGE. See how easy it is!

I like to grocery shop and meal prep on Sundays. My weeks are usually crazy busy (pun intended). I wake up 2 hours before I have to leave for work. This allows me time to make my breakfast, get in my workout, clean up, pack my lunch tote with my meals for the day that have already been prepared, and get out the door. If I had to do more than put meals together, if I had to cook food to take with me each and every day, I'd have to wake up even earlier, which would mean I was shorting myself on sleep. Sleep is also very important to losing weight like crazy. But, since I've already grocery shopped and meal prepped, I can get my sleep, have my breakfast, get in my 30-minute workout, shower and get ready for the day, and get out of the house on time. Being prepared allows me to stay on point with my nutrition and my fitness.

If you would like to see a demo of exactly how I meal prep, as well as how to do it if you do want to cook and prepare all of your meals for the week, you can find those videos in *Ultimate Portion Fix*.

Tip Get More Sleep

Remember what I said at the beginning about not "sleeping" on these crazy easy tips, unless the tip was to get more sleep? Well here it is: GET MORE SLEEP. Our bodies need time to rest, recover, and repair from the day, especially if you are exercising each day. Sleep is where the magic happens. Most people think the magic of working out happens during the workout; it doesn't. The workout is where you tear your muscle fibers on a microscopic level. Don't worry, this is normal. When you sleep is when the muscle repairs itself, ultimately making it stronger. Lack of sleep can also lead to stronger cravings the next day. When you're tired, your body can start to crave sugar more. That's because it's looking for a readily available energy source, and your body is smart; it knows that sugar is just a quick hit. That's why it's sometimes referred to as a sugar rush. If we want to help those cravings subside, then we need to get more sleep. Aim for at least 8 hours a night.

STEP 6 Track Your Containers

Last, but certainly not least, we need to track our containers. This is HUGE to your success. You know how many of each container you get a day, and you know which containers you are combining at each meal, but it's very easy to forget halfway through the day what you've already had if you aren't tracking them in your phone, on the app, or at least on a piece of paper. Tracking your containers ensures that you don't overeat or undereat on your containers.

LET'S REVIEW:

That's it for the *Lose Weight Like Crazy* plan. We still have a few things to cover, to make sure you are getting the most out of this plan, but first, let's review the 6 basic steps for losing weight like crazy even if you have a crazy life.

STEP 1: Identify your "WHY."

STEP 2: Decide whether or not you are exercising regularly with this plan, and determine your calorie range.

STEP 3: Find your calorie bracket, and see how many of each container you get a day.

STEP 4: Make a meal plan for the week.

STEP 5: Grocery shop and meal prep, so you set yourself up for success.

STEP 6: Track your containers.

Things to ADD IN:	Things to TAKE OUT:
• Exercise	• Excuses
• Water	• Soda
• Variety of Fruits & Vegetables	• Milkshakes disguised as coffee
• Self-love	• Highly processed foods
• Sleep	

Things to have in MODERATION:

• Dessert   • Alcohol

FREQUENTLY ASKED QUESTIONS

This is a lot of food; do I have to eat all of my containers in a day?

Yes, it can seem like a lot of food when you are first getting used to this way of eating. The foods you are eating are nutrient-dense but lower in calories than most junk food. That means you get to eat more of it. Your body does need a certain amount of fuel, just to function. The *Lose Weight Like Crazy* plan has you at a big enough caloric deficit for you to lose weight but still remain healthy and give your body all the support it needs to function properly. If you don't eat all of your containers, you will end up at an even bigger deficit, and this can actually slow your body's weight loss. Too big of a deficit, and your body will hold on tight to everything you give it, to make sure it has enough fuel for survival.

For those people that are eating in plans E and F, it is a lot of food, and it can be hard to eat all of it in the beginning. I definitely don't want you feeling so full that you feel sick, so if you absolutely cannot stomach all of the food you are supposed to be eating, then it's important to know what you can reduce. If you feel like you can't eat any more, you can't just say, "I'm not eating any more vegetables," which seems to be what people want to do. If you can't eat any more, you can skip 1 RED container. If you still can't finish all the food, you can skip 1 YELLOW container, and finally, if you still can't eat any more, you can skip 1 GREEN. This is only for plans E and F.

Before you cut out any of your containers, I'm going to encourage you to look at the foods that you are choosing. This is where tracking comes into play. Are you picking a lot of foods that sit really heavy and are harder to digest? Things like red meat, potatoes or cruciferous vegetables? If so, can you change it up and pick fish or chicken? Maybe try mixed greens for some of your vegetables. This is also where having Shakeology can really help. Shakeology mixed with water counts as 1 RED container (protein), but you can blend in frozen fruit to add a PURPLE, or frozen cauliflower for a GREEN. You can even add in 1 tsp of nut butter to count as 1 of your tsps. This can help you fit in containers without leaving you feeling overly full.

What do I do if I miss a container?

Tracking your containers in this book, in your phone, on the Beachbody app, or with a printed tracker sheet should help prevent you from missing a container, but no one is perfect. We all slip up at some point. If you accidentally miss a container in a day, it's not the end of the world. You don't actually need to do anything. Just pick back up the next day, and keep moving forward. However, if you notice that you are consistently forgetting containers, then it's time to take a different approach to how you've been keeping track, or to start tracking if you haven't been doing it.

What do I do if I overeat on my containers?

In an ideal world you'll be keeping track and sticking to the plan, but once again, a slipup happens from time to time, even with the best of intentions. If you happen to go over on a fruit or a vegetable, it's not the end of the world, but pay attention to what was going on that allowed for this to happen. Did you overeat because you were still hungry? Did you go over on your containers because you weren't paying attention? Or, did you go over because of an emotional reason? This tends to be where the biggest slipups happen, and it's usually with the coveted YELLOW container. You do great all day, stick to the plan, and then something happens. You have a fight with your significant other, you have a challenging day at work, your friends call and want to go out for drinks, and before you know it, that plan you were doing so well with all day goes out the window. Your results are entirely up to you. I can and have given you all the tools you need to lose weight like crazy, but you have to be in charge of you. You have to be responsible for what you choose to put into your body. The plan is designed for you to be able to have a cocktail (approved from the list above or from the *FIXATE* cooking show, and books) but you have to sub it in. That means if you get 3 YELLOWS in a day and you want a glass of wine at the end of the day, then you will only eat 2 carbohydrates from the YELLOW list, and the last YELLOW will be your 5-ounce glass of wine.

Slipups happen, but if they happen regularly, you need to take a deeper look at what's going on. Go back to what I talked about in the beginning of the book. Are you processing your emotions in a healthy way? Do you have a support system around you that you can lean on when you need it? Did you define a strong enough "WHY?" If you need more support, I'm always here. You can sign up to be a part of my Monthly Fix group. To learn more visit TeamACPortionFix.com.

Is it OK to eat the same thing every day?

There is something to be said for having some consistency from day to day with your meals. It makes grocery shopping and meal prepping that much easier. BUT, this is important, you don't want to eat the same thing day in and day out for weeks on end. First, it will get boring and could lead to you falling off track. Second, and more importantly, your body needs a variety of vitamins, minerals, and nutrients. If you eat the same 2 or 3 vegetables, fruits, or carbohydrates every single day, then you're probably not going to get a wide variety of nutrients. My best advice is to switch it up from week to week.

How can I speed up my weight loss even more?

This plan is designed for you to lose weight like crazy; all you have to do is follow it. To get the best-of-the-best results, try eating

"I no longer feel sluggish and disconnected!"

—Kourtney D, 37, Independent Team Beachbody Coach, Armonk, NY

Kourtney D., a teacher and married mother of 2, missed the confident, energetic woman she once was. After having her children 2 years apart, she found herself using every bit of energy just to keep up and care for 2 kids under age 3.

"I was tired and felt defeated," Kourtney says. "I was alive, but not living."

Although she felt intimidated to start a fitness and nutrition program, Kourtney faced her fears and jumped into my *21 Day Fix* program. Her goal: Lose 15 pounds in 21 days.

"I hit it and was overjoyed," Kourtney says. The lifestyle change was just what she needed.

"I totally used to skip meals. I would often go all day without eating and just sip on a cup of coffee instead. I thought that if I starved myself then I would lose weight. This program taught me that you need to fuel your body right if you want to speed

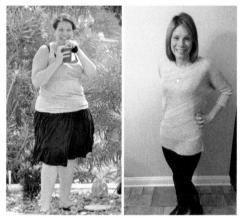

Day 1: 198 lbs.   Day 210*: 134 lbs.

up your metabolism and lose weight."

Kourtney weighed 198 pounds when she started following my workouts and using my portion control containers. "I will use the containers for the rest of my life; I view them as the new food pyramid," she says. After completing 10 consecutive rounds, Kourtney lost 64 pounds and feels great at a healthy weight of 134.

"I am a better mom, wife, friend, and now coach!"

from the top third of each of the food lists for at least 85% to 90% of your meals. Make sure you're tracking your containers and not overeating or undereating on them. To get the absolute best, fastest results, limit treats/substitutions. I've taught you how to include desserts and alcohol in the plan and still lose weight, but if you're looking to speed things up, cutting these things out for a while is a great way to do it. Last, but not least, be patient with your body. Unfortunately, it's much easier to gain weight than it is to lose it. While you can gain 3 to 5 pounds in one weekend with poor nutrition, chances are you won't lose those same 5 pounds with one weekend of proper nutrition. Stay the course, trust the process, and watch your body lose weight like crazy.

How do I break through a plateau?

This is probably one of the biggest questions I get. Before I give you advice for breaking through a plateau, we need to actually define what a plateau is. Not losing weight for 1 or even 2 weeks does not count as a plateau. Also, the number on the scale is not the only thing that determines if you have truly hit a plateau.

Let me explain what happens. You start a new healthy way of eating and exercising and you're eating fewer calories than your body is burning. That means you're eating at a caloric deficit. This starts the initial weight-loss process. Hopefully, you're exercising on top of that, which is not only contributing to a caloric burn, it's building lean muscle, which helps give you a nice, sculpted look. In the first week of following this plan, I've seen people lose anywhere from 2 to 10 pounds, depending on the amount of weight they have to lose. Keep in mind, the more weight you have to lose, the more weight you're likely to lose at the beginning of this process, when it is the biggest shock to your system.

Let's look at a hypothetical example:

Mary is 5'4" and weighs 180 pounds. She eats a poor diet of fairly processed foods and soda, and she works a 9-to-5 desk job. Mary decides to follow the *Lose Weight Like Crazy* nutrition plan and incorporates the workouts from this book. In the first week, she's feeling good and drops 5 pounds! Mary is beyond excited and motivated to keep going. She stays on point with her nutrition and workouts for the second week in a row. At the end of the second week, she steps on the scale, expecting to see another 5 pounds gone, but this week she loses only 1 pound. Instantly, Mary is mad. She starts to second-guess the plan, wondering why it worked so well in the first week and not the second. Now, she starts to repeat a negative story in her mind: "See, I knew nothing would work for me in the long run. Why even bother?" That way of thinking is a big mistake and stops so many people in their tracks before they ever even truly get started. What Mary doesn't know, probably because she's never been taught, is that this is a very normal response for the body. When your body lets go of a large amount of weight in a short period of time (yes, 5 pounds in a week is a lot to your body), it will take a "pause for the cause," as I like to say. Your body is very smart. It's not used to losing 5 pounds in one week. That is a signal to your body that something might be wrong. So, it "pauses." It goes into a full "systems check." Your body is protecting itself. It needs to make sure there isn't a major problem, like famine. If your body lost 5 pounds a week for multiple weeks in a row, this could be very taxing on your organs and your body as a whole. So, it slows the process down for a minute, to make sure everything is OK. Once it realizes that everything is, in fact, OK, that you are not starving, that a steady supply of fuel is coming in, it will continue to let go of excess weight. But that can't ever happen if you give up in the first week or 2.

Another time people tend to think they have hit a plateau is when they are down to those last, stubborn 5 to 10 pounds. Again, if your body has let go of a large amount of weight in a short period of time, it might take a little longer for those last few pounds to come off, but if you stay the course, they will. This is usually the time where you need to dial it in a little more. A true plateau has happened when you still have weight to lose, but you are not losing weight, or inches, or gaining any more strength, meaning you're not able to lift heavier or last longer in a workout.

If all 3 of these things are happening—not losing weight inches or gaining strength/endurance—then we need to look at a few things. First is your nutrition: Are you eating from the top third of the food lists for at least 85% to 90% of your meals? Are you drinking enough water? Are you getting enough sleep? How hard are you pushing in your workouts? Could you lift a little heavier, push a little harder, go a little longer, do a little more? Our bodies adapt to stress over time. That is what exercise is, it's a stressor on the body. It's a good stress, but stress nonetheless. If your body has adapted to the workout that you are doing, you won't continue to see as much progress as when it was new and unfamiliar to your body. So, change it up. This is why I have 8 different workout programs on Beachbody On Demand. If you're ready to switch it up, I highly recommend trying one of them. There is something for everyone: cardio, weight training, endurance training, Pilates, yoga, and even dance.

Even if your body does hit a plateau, it's no reason to quit what you are doing. The only way you truly stop making progress is by quitting. What happens if you give up? That won't help you lose the last 5 to 10 pounds either. Chances are, you might even start to backslide into old, bad habits. So instead of getting frustrated, ask yourself what else you can do to take care of your body and give it what it needs.

Push Through a Plateau with My Top 10 Tips

1. Cut out treats for 3 weeks
2. Cut out alcohol for 3 weeks
3. Eat from the top third of the food lists
4. Change up the foods that you are eating. Try new fruits, vegetables, and carbohydrates
5. Drink half of your body weight in ounces of water a day
6. Try pushing a little harder in your workouts
7. Change up your workout program
8. Change up the time of day you are exercising (little changes can still help shock your system)
9. Make sure you are getting at least 8 hours of sleep a night
10. Practice self-care and de-stressing

Can I drop down a bracket to lose weight even faster?

Absolutely NOT. Don't try to outsmart the science behind the program. This method is tried-and-true. It's worked for hundreds of thousands of people, and it can work for you, too, if you follow it the way I have it written. The formula I provided already puts you at a caloric deficit. The deficit is big enough to help you lose weight like crazy, but not so big that it will have the exact opposite effect. Your body needs a certain amount of fuel to function. Give it too little, and it will hold on to every last little bit, to make sure it has the energy it needs to perform all of its tasks. It requires energy to breathe, to keep your heart beating, to digest, to pump blood, to excrete waste, to just be awake. You don't want to starve your body. If you don't follow the plan the way I have it written, then you aren't actually following my plan that's proven to work, and I can't say what kind of results you can or can't expect because I only know THIS plan and how it works. Trust the process and stick to it.

How to Survive Eating Out and Special Occasions
and Still Lose Weight Like Crazy

MY TOP 10 TIPS FOR EATING OUT

1. If you know where you will be going out to eat, look at the menu online to get an idea of what you might like to have.

2. If you do get a chance to look at the menu ahead of time, make sure you save containers for the meal that you would like to have. If you don't get a chance to look at a menu ahead of time, then I always recommend saving at least 1 RED, 1 YELLOW, 1 GREEN and 2 tsps. I say 2 tsps because restaurants tend to cook with more oil than you would at home.

3. If you know you are going to have an alcoholic beverage or a dessert, save swaps for them. Remember, you only get a total of 3 swaps for the week. Avoid the cocktails that are loaded with juices or other mixers. Keep it clean and simple, a clear alcohol mixed with soda water is best. You can ask them to muddle it with fresh herbs or fruit to add more flavor. If you do fruit, you need to account for that with your containers. Most desserts are much bigger than 1 serving, and would probably be closer to 2 or more YELLOW containers, so if you're going to enjoy dessert, maybe get one for the table to share, or take a few bites and leave the rest.

4. If you haven't saved any swaps for alcohol or dessert, you can have a soda water with lemon and lime to enjoy while others have a cocktail, and you could order a cup of coffee or tea to sip on at the end of the meal, instead of overindulging in dessert.

5. Don't go out to eat famished. When you do, this is when your eyes become bigger than your stomach. Suddenly, everything sounds delicious, and you "need" an appetizer, entrée, and dessert.

6. Say no to bread. Often restaurants will bring bread to the table as soon as you sit down. If you haven't shown up hungry, you can politely decline the bread basket all-together. If you have decided you want to have bread, make sure you save a YELLOW container for it. Take the one piece that you are going to have and then send the basket away.

7. When possible, order off of the appetizer menu. These portions tend to be more in line with a real serving size compared to bigger entrées.

8. If you know entrée sizes are large, you can either split it with whomever you are going out to eat or when your entrée arrives, you can immediately ask for a box. Box half of it up to take home for another meal so you don't overeat at one sitting.

9. Avoid ordering things that are described as fried, cheesy, breaded, creamy, melted, smothered, or crispy.

10. Don't be afraid to order what you want and how you want it. I know this one can be challenging. We don't want to be a pain in the butt, asking for food to be prepared a certain way that might not be listed on the menu. Here's the thing: it's your body and you're paying for the food, so order how you want it. If you want easy oil or no oil, ASK FOR IT. If you want something baked instead of fried. ASK FOR IT. If you want your dressing on the side, ASK FOR IT. We have to stop feeling bad for asking for our food the way we want it to be. I waited tables for 15 years; as long as you do it politely, it's OK.

Surviving Special Occasions

One of the biggest things that can throw people off of their weight-loss journey, or stop them from even starting, is a holiday. There are countless holidays to celebrate throughout the year, Memorial Day, Fourth of July, Labor Day, Halloween, Thanksgiving, Christmas, Hanukkah, New Year's Eve, New Year's Day, Super Bowl (to some it's a holiday), Valentine's Day, Easter, Passover, Cinco De Mayo, birthday, yours, your friends', your family members', the list goes on and on. Is there a month in the year without something to celebrate? Probably not. So, if you're waiting for "the holidays" to be over to start eating better, you'll be waiting forever. If you're using, "it's a holiday," to throw caution to the wind when it comes to staying on track with your healthy eating, then you'll forever be falling off track. Instead of using holidays as an excuse to overindulge, and even downright gorge yourself on food that isn't good for you, let's look at ways that we can enjoy the holidays while still staying completely on track. It's usually from Halloween to New Year's Day that is the hardest time to stay focused and on point, with the number of holidays and parties that happen during this time of year, but these tips work for any and all holidays.

MY TOP 10 TIPS FOR SURVIVING SPECIAL OCCASIONS

1. Make sure you're getting your workouts in.

You might have expected me to start with a nutrition tip, but I'm starting with a fitness tip for a reason. In my 15+ years of working in the health industry, here is what I've observed. On the days people get their workouts in, they tend to eat better. For whatever reason, the day they skip a workout also seems to be the day they let loose with their nutrition, as well. It seems so counterintuitive to me. If I don't get a workout in, I try to be even better about my nutrition, but for some reason, this is not the norm. So, make sure you're getting your workouts in. Not just on the holiday, but for that week. Don't let the holiday week be the week you slack on your workouts. Getting that extra calorie burn in can keep you not only feeling good, but it can also keep you in the mindset of not wanting to undo all of your hard work by eating poorly.

2. Don't go to a holiday celebration hungry.

I see people do this all the time. Take Thanksgiving, for instance. They get excited that there will be a feast later in the day, so they wait the entire day to eat, so that they can really indulge in that Thanksgiving meal. You might think this is the best answer—save all your containers for that one meal—but remember, part of the plan is practicing portion control and not overfilling your stomach in any one sitting. It's OK to save a few extra containers (probably YELLOWS and tsps.) for that meal, but it's important to still eat throughout the day leading up to the meal. This way you won't overeat.

3. Save your treats.

It's important to be able to enjoy life and food with family and friends, and not obsess about whether one meal is going to ruin all of your hard work. You don't want to feel like a total outsider with your family and friends, either. The good news is, you don't have to. You can have 2 to 3 treats/swaps in a week. If you have a special occasion that you're celebrating and you're going to want to have a few glasses of wine, or wine and dessert, make sure you save your swaps for this. I don't typically recommend saving them all for one night, but in the instance of a holiday, I do. For example, you're going to Thanksgiving dinner, and you know you want a glass of wine with dinner and pumpkin pie after, save all 3 swaps for this. If you are in plan B, you get 3 YELLOW containers a day. That means you won't have any other "treats" during the week, and on Thanksgiving Day, instead of having your normal 3 YELLOW containers, you would only have your glass of wine and your small slice of pumpkin pie. If it's store-bought pumpkin pie, I would count that as 2 YELLOWS. If it's a *FIXATE* recipe, then you would use the container count given. Now, if you're in a higher plan, like plan D, you still only get 2 to 3 swaps for the week, but you get 4 YELLOW containers in a day. That means you could have your glass of wine, your slice of pumpkin pie, and you could have one other YELLOW container that day. If you need more help understanding treats/swaps, check out my video in *Ultimate Portion Fix* on Beachbody On Demand.

4. Make a recipe that's a part of your plan.

Most people think healthy eating has to be boring or bland. If you have tried any of the recipes in this book, or any of the 300+ recipes in my cookbooks and on my cooking show, *FIXATE*, then you know that couldn't be further from the truth. If you're hosting a holiday meal, you could make the entire menu from *FIXATE*. We have included recipes for just about every occasion there is, and we have entrées, side dishes, soups, salads, and desserts. I typically suggest NOT telling your friends and family up front that the meal is "healthy." Not because I'm encouraging you to be deceitful, but because people have preconceived notions of "healthy" food. Instead, cook and serve, and once everyone tells you how delicious the meal was, you can tell them that it was all a part of your *Lose Weight Like Crazy* plan, and they can feel really good about everything they just ate. If you're not hosting the event, but instead going to someone else's house, offer to bring a dish. At least there will be one thing there that you know was made healthy and is on plan for you. I typically like to bring one of the yummy *FIXATE* salads because it guarantees I will get a vegetable serving at the meal, and I know I can eat a little extra to fill me up, instead of eating all the other heavy food that might be served. The same thing holds true if you are going to a potluck. Bring a dish that you know is approved and that you've saved containers for.

5. Don't go back for seconds.

Why is it that on the holidays we act like we haven't had a meal in months? Suddenly, it's OK to fill your plate until food is practically falling off AND we go back for seconds and thirds?! Do you do this with dinner on a random Tuesday? I'm guessing not. If you do, it's time to stop. The amount of food that fits on a dinner plate is more than enough for one sitting, and while the food might be delicious, tempting you to go back for more, you need to stop and ask yourself, "Am I still actually hungry?" If the answer is no, which it probably is, then you don't need more. At this point, you would be eating purely for pleasure, not for fuel. I'm trying to teach you to change the mentality around continuing to eat even when you are not hungry. Put on your plate what you intend to have for that meal (what you have containers for), sit down with it, be present, enjoy your food, taste your food, chew your food, don't just inhale your food. Make it an experience, and when you're finished with what is on your plate, that's it, you're finished. Clear your plate, and move on to something else.

6. Only eat the foods you really love.

Holiday celebrations tend to have multiple protein dishes, multiple carbohydrate dishes, even multiple vegetable dishes. Choose only the foods you REALLY want, and put those on your plate. Thanksgiving dinner at my family's house always has pasta, potatoes, and stuffing. Even though I get 3 YELLOWS in a day, eating them all at one meal would make me feel very full. Instead, I pick the one that I want the most: that's stuffing. I also pick this because I tend to make pasta and potatoes throughout the year, but I only make stuffing on Thanksgiving. Your other option would be to have a half-serving of 2 of the items. So, maybe you fill your YELLOW container halfway full with pasta, put that on your plate, and then fill it halfway full with stuffing and put that on your plate. This way you get to taste both dishes but still only have 1 YELLOW serving.

7. Use a smaller plate.

Instead of using a 12-in. or 16-in. dinner plate, use a smaller appetizer plate. Using a bigger plate can make you feel like you need to put more food on it to have a "full" serving, when in fact, you've put more than 1 serving on the plate. By using a smaller plate, you limit the amount of food that will fit on it, and thus have more appropriate-sized portions. You can also start by putting your vegetables on your plate. Your vegetable serving is 1 cup. By putting that on first, you've already taken up a nice-sized portion of the plate. Next, put your protein, and put your carbohydrate on last, when there is the least amount of room.

8. Leave the leftovers.

At the end of the day, enjoying one meal, even if it's not the healthiest, really shouldn't undo all of your hard work. But, eat that same meal for a few days in a row, and that's a different story. Let's continue using Thanksgiving dinner as our example. Let's say you go to your aunt's house for Thanksgiving, and she cooks the entire meal. You know she's using lots of butter, sugar, and salt in the cooking. There are multiple kinds of potatoes, meat, bread, and dessert, and you decide to try all of it. First of all, there's only so much you can eat before you're going to start to feel sick. So, you eat the meal and enjoy the meal. Totally fine. But then your aunt says, "I made you a plate to take home." This plate has 2 to 3 more servings of every single dish. You take it home, and over the next few days, you continue to eat Thanksgiving dinner. Houston, we have a problem. This is where it becomes excessive, and this is where it can throw you off track. You don't need to eat Thanksgiving dinner all weekend long, so when your aunt or anyone else offers leftovers, politely decline. Now, on the flip side of that, if you're the one who made the big Thanksgiving dinner, hopefully you used your *FIX-ATE* recipes to do it, so if you wanted to eat it more than once over the weekend, you could. But if you didn't, then send family and friends home with leftovers. That way it's not sitting in your fridge, tempting you or making you feel like you are wasting food.

9. Don't have your conversations at the buffet table, or standing around the food in general.

It's one thing to enjoy conversation with your family and friends once you've put food on your plate and sat down at the table to eat, but it's another to stand at the buffet or snack table and do it. Often when we stand around a table full of food, having a conversation, we snack. We have a handful of this, a bite of that, a taste of this, just a few more chips, never really paying attention to what or how much we are eating. This is a fast track to eating way more than you should and not staying within your allotted containers. Instead, put the food you want to eat on your plate, while being mindful of it, then move your conversation away from the buffet.

10. Hydrate.

We've talked a lot about the importance of being hydrated. I'm talking about it a little differently here. When you're at a celebration, it's easy to get a little carried away with the adult beverages. In order to slow your consumption down, have one 8-ounce glass of water in between your alcoholic beverages. Not only will this slow down how much you drink at the celebration, it will help keep you hydrated, so you don't wake up with a nasty headache the next morning.

CRAZY EASY, CRAZY DELICIOUS!

23 Mouthwatering Recipes to Get You Started on Your Journey to Lose Weight Like Crazy.

Created by professional chef, co-host of my cooking show *FIXATE* & my brother, Bobby Calabrese

Recipes containing the **GF** icon are designed to be Gluten-Free and contain no gluten. If you are following a gluten-free diet, remember to check all labels to confirm your ingredients are 100% gluten-free, since foods are often processed at facilities that also process wheat and other grains.

Recipes containing the **V** icon are designed to be Vegan and contain no animal products. Please read product labels for each ingredient to ensure this to be the case.

Recipes containing the **VG** icon are designed to be Lacto-Ovo vegetarian and contain no poultry, meat, or fish. Please read product labels for each ingredient to ensure this to be the case.

Blueberry Pie Oats

Serves: 1 (approx. 2 cups)   **Prep Time:** 15 min. + overnight   **Cooking Time:** None

Container Equivalents (per serving): ■1 ■½ ▪2 ▪½ ●—1

For Oats:

1 cup	fresh blueberries, divided use
½ cup	unsweetened coconut milk beverage
1 tsp.	pure maple syrup
¼ cup	dry rolled oats
1 Tbsp.	chia seeds
¼ cup + 2 Tbsp.	reduced-fat (2%) plain Greek yogurt

For Crumble Topping:

2 Tbsp.	coarsely crushed graham crackers, gluten-free
1 tsp.	extra-virgin coconut oil
1 pinch	sea salt (or Himalayan salt)

1. Place a medium saucepan over medium-high heat. Add ¾ cup blueberries, coconut milk, and maple syrup; bring to a simmer.

2. Stir in oats and chia seeds. Cook 5 minutes, stirring often, until oats are cooked and liquid is absorbed; remove from heat.

3. Stir in yogurt and remaining ¼ cup blueberries.

4. Transfer to a sealed container; allow to cool. Refrigerate overnight or until chilled.

5. For the crumble topping, place crushed graham crackers, coconut oil, and salt in a medium mixing bowl; mix well with clean hands. Cover and set aside until ready to serve.

6. When ready to serve, sprinkle crumble topping onto oat mixture; enjoy!

Nutrition Information (per serving): Calories: 392 / Total Fat: 16 g / Saturated Fat: 9 g / Cholesterol: 9 mg / Sodium: 345 mg / Carbohydrates: 52 g / Fiber: 12 g / Sugars: 23 g / Protein: 16 g

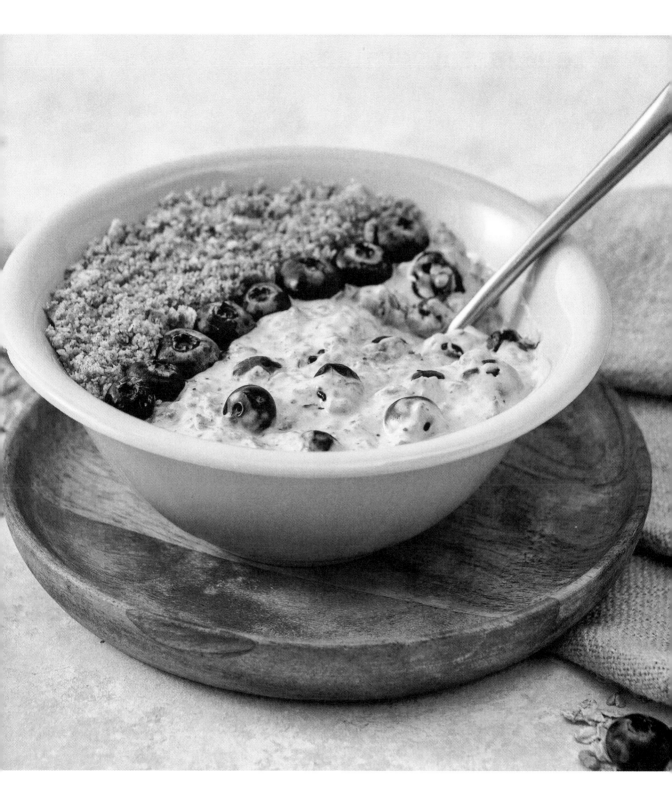

Breakfast Enchiladas

Serves: 4 (1 enchilada each)   **Prep Time:** 15 min.   **Cooking Time:** 45 min.

Container Equivalents (per serving): ⬛1 ⬛1 ⬜1 ⬛1 🥄1

1 Tbsp.	extra-virgin olive oil
1 cup	chopped onion (approx. 1⅓ medium)
1 cup	chopped green bell pepper (approx. 1⅓ medium)
2	cloves garlic, finely chopped
1¼ cups	chopped tomato (approx. 2¼ medium)
1 tsp.	chili powder
½ tsp.	sea salt (or Himalayan salt), divided use
4	(6-inch) whole-grain tortillas
6 slices	ham (nitrate- and nitrite-free), chopped
1 cup	shredded cheddar jack cheese, divided use
4	large eggs
1 cup	unsweetened soy milk
2 tsp.	all-purpose flour
2 slices	turkey bacon, cooked, crumbled
½ cup	sliced green onion (approx. 4 medium stalks)
¼ cup	chopped fresh cilantro

Special Equipment:

Nonstick cooking spray

Aluminum foil

1. Preheat oven to 350°F.

2. Lightly coat medium baking dish with spray; set aside.

3. Heat olive oil in a large skillet over medium-high heat until fragrant. Add onion, bell pepper, garlic, tomato, chili powder, and ¼ tsp. salt. Cook for 5 to 7 minutes, until bell peppers are tender and tomatoes have broken down into a sauce.

4. Fill each tortilla with a quarter of the onion mixture, a quarter of the chopped ham, and 2 Tbsp. cheese. Roll them up and place, seam-side down, in a 9-in. x 9-in. baking dish.

5. Place eggs, soy milk, flour, and remaining ¼ tsp. salt in a medium mixing bowl; whisk to combine. Pour egg mixture over enchiladas.

6. Top enchiladas with remaining ¼ cup cheese, bacon, and green onion; cover with aluminum foil and bake for 35 minutes. Remove foil; continue baking an additional 10 minutes until eggs are set.

7. Serve an enchilada on each of 4 plates. Divide cilantro evenly among each enchilada and enjoy!

Recipe Note:

- To prep these enchiladas in advance, pour the egg mixture over the enchiladas, then cover with aluminum foil and refrigerate overnight. Preheat oven, then proceed to step 6 when ready to bake.

Nutritional Information (per serving): Calories: 413 / Total Fat: 22 g / Saturated Fat: 7 g / Cholesterol: 270 mg / Sodium: 1,464 mg / Carbohydrates: 25 g / Fiber: 11 g / Sugars: 5 g / Protein: 28 g

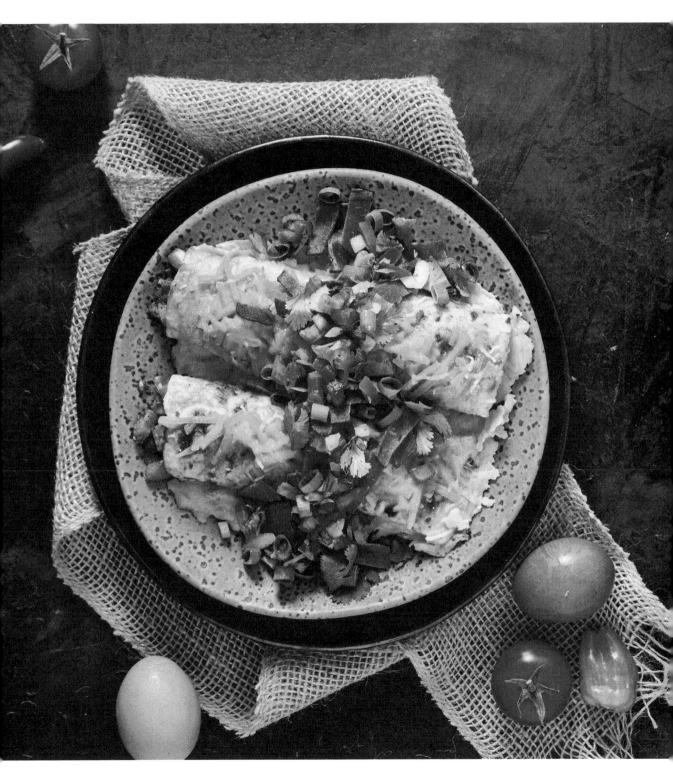

GF

Slow-Cooker Sausage and Egg Grits

Serves: 4 (approx. ¾ cup each)   **Prep Time:** 15 min.   **Cooking Time:** 8 hrs.
Container Equivalents (per serving):   ■ 1   ■ 1   ■ ½   ●—1

1 Tbsp.	ghee (organic grass-fed, if possible)
1½ cups	*FIXATE* Breakfast Sausage
½ cup	stone-ground grits
¼ tsp.	sea salt (or Himalayan salt)
2 cups	water
4	large eggs, lightly beaten
½ cup	shredded cheddar cheese

Special Equipment:

Nonstick cooking spray

1. Place ghee in a large skillet; heat over high heat until very hot.

2. Add sausage and cook until browned; transfer to a slow cooker.

3. Add grits, salt, and water to slow cooker; cover and cook on low for 8 hours, until grits are tender and creamy.

4. When grits are done, place a nonstick pan, lightly coated with spray, over medium heat. Add eggs and cook, stirring occasionally, for 3 to 6 minutes, or until eggs are set.

5. Stir eggs and cheese into grits mixture.

6. Divide evenly among 4 plates. Enjoy!

FIXATE Breakfast Sausage

1 lb.	raw 93% lean ground turkey,
2 Tbsp.	pure maple syrup,
1½ tsp.	sea salt (or Himalayan salt),
1 tsp.	finely chopped fresh sage,
1 tsp.	finely chopped fresh rosemary,
¼ tsp.	ground black pepper,
¼ tsp.	ground nutmeg,
1 dash	ground juniper berries,
2 tsp.	ice cold water

1. Combine all ingredients in a large mixing bowl; mix with clean hands until just blended. (Do not overmix, as that will make the sausage tough.) Set aside.

2. Heat 1 tsp. extra-virgin olive oil in large nonstick skillet over medium-high heat.

3. Add turkey mixture; cook, stirring frequently to break turkey into crumble-sized pieces, for 5 to 8 minutes, or until turkey is no longer pink.

Recipe Note:

- It makes 4 (¾-cup) servings and can be stored in an airtight container in the refrigerator for 3 days, or in the freezer for up to 3 months.

Nutrition Information (per serving): Calories: 310 / Total Fat: 17 g / Saturated Fat: 7 g / Cholesterol: 260 mg / Sodium: 730 mg / Carbohydrates: 18 g. / Fiber: 1 g / Sugars: 3 g / Protein: 21 g

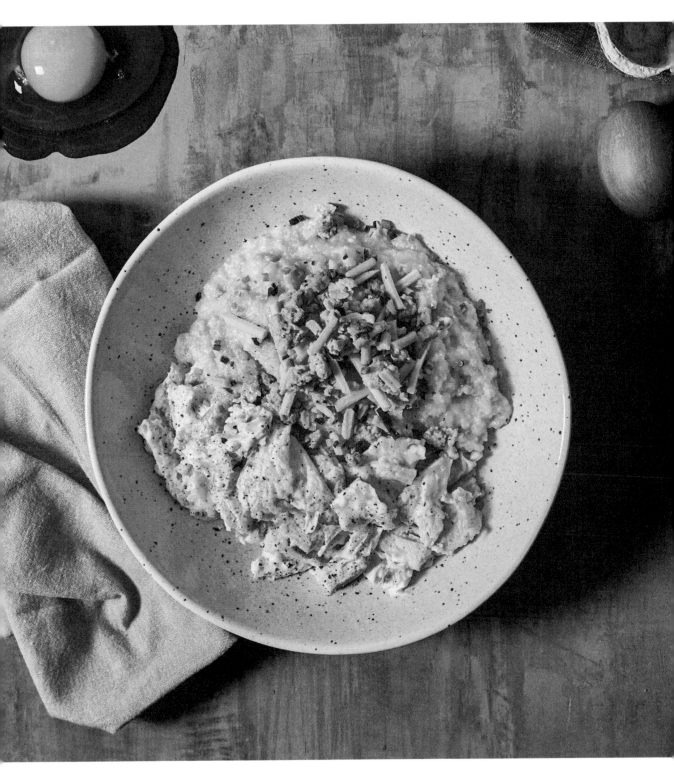

Cajun Sausage and Apple Skillet

GF

Serves: 4 (approx. 1 cup each) **Prep Time:** 10 min. **Cooking Time:** 15 min.
Container Equivalents (per serving): ⬛ 1 ⬛ ½ ⬛ 1 🥄 1

1 lb.	raw low-fat turkey andouille sausage
1 Tbsp.	ghee (organic grass-fed, if possible)
3 cups	shredded green cabbage
¾ cup	chopped onion (approx. 1 medium)
3	cloves garlic, finely chopped
2 Tbsp.	cider vinegar
2 cups	peeled, chopped apple
1 Tbsp.	Cajun seasoning
½ tsp.	sea salt (or Himalayan salt)
¼ cup	sliced green onion (approx. 2 medium stalks)

1. Remove the sausage from the casing (if your sausage did not come in casing, skip this step).

2. Heat ghee in a large cast-iron or heavy-bottomed skillet over medium-high heat. Add sausage; cook, stirring occasionally, for 5 minutes, until browned. Remove to a plate using a slotted spoon.

3. Add cabbage, onion, garlic, and vinegar; cook for 3 to 5 minutes, until cabbage is tender-crisp.

4. Return sausage to pan; add apple, Cajun seasoning, and salt. Cook for 2 to 3 minutes, until apples are tender.

5. Garnish with green onion and serve.

Nutrition Information (per serving): Calories: 264 / Total Fat: 14 g / Saturated Fat: 5 g / Cholesterol: 97 mg / Sodium: 1,404 mg / Carbohydrates: 17 g / Fiber: 4 g / Sugars: 10 g / Protein: 20 g

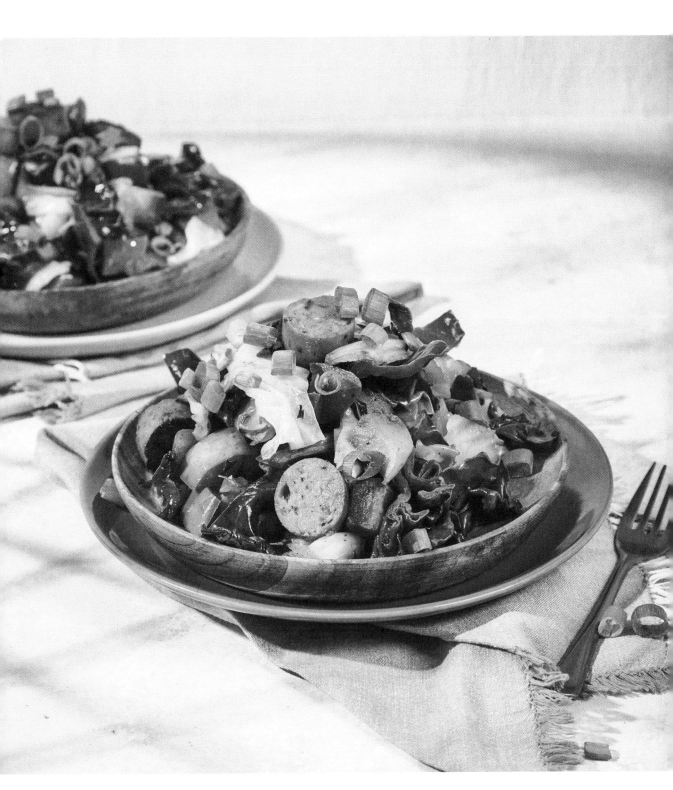

Curry Chicken Salad

Serves: 4 (approx. 1¼ cups each) **Prep Time:** 15 min. **Cooking Time:** None
Container Equivalents (per serving): ■ ½ ■ ½ ■ 1 ■ 1

3 cups	chopped cooked chicken breast, skinless, boneless
1 cup	chopped green apple
1 cup	halved seedless red grapes
½ cup	chopped celery (approx. 1 medium stalk)
½ cup	thinly sliced red onion (approx. ½ medium)
½ cup	sliced green onion (approx. 4 medium stalks)
¼ cup	finely chopped fresh dill weed
¼ cup	finely chopped fresh tarragon
¼ cup	pine nuts
¼ cup	reduced-fat (2%) plain Greek yogurt
2 Tbsp.	fresh lemon juice
1 Tbsp.	mayonnaise
1 Tbsp.	curry powder
½ tsp.	sea salt (or Himalayan salt)

- Place chicken, apple, grapes, celery, red onion, green onion, dill, tarragon, pine nuts, yogurt, lemon juice, mayonnaise, curry powder, and salt in a large mixing bowl. Gently fold until thoroughly combined.

Nutrition Information (per serving:) Calories: 297 / Total Fat: 12 g / Saturated Fat: 2 g / Cholesterol: 86 mg / Sodium: 386 mg / Carbohydrates: 17 g / Fiber: 3 g / Sugars: 12 g / Protein: 29 g

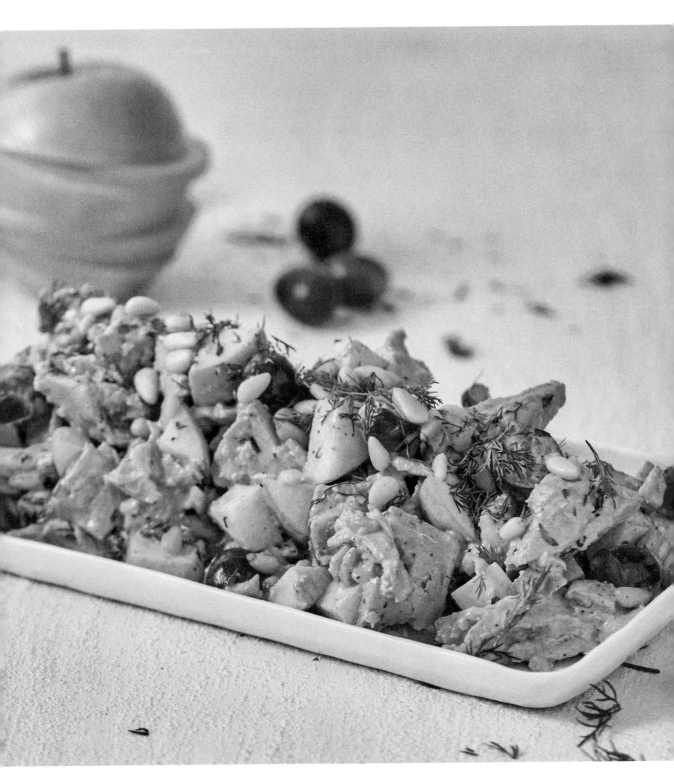

Crispy Tofu Buddha Bowl GF V VG

Serves: 1 (approx. 2½ cups)   **Prep Time:** 10 min.   **Cooking Time:** 10 min.
Container Equivalents (per serving): ■ 1½ ■ ½ ■ 1 ■ 1½ ●— 1
Vegan Container Equivalents (per serving): ■ 1½ ■ ½ ■ ½ A 1 B ½ ●— 1

For Sauce:

1 Tbsp.	reduced-sodium tamari soy sauce
1½ tsp.	coconut sugar
1 pinch	garlic powder
1 pinch	ground ginger
1 pinch	curry powder

For Bowl:

1 tsp.	cornstarch (preferably GMO-free)
4 oz.	firm tofu, drained, patted dry
1 tsp.	sesame oil
1 cup	baby bok choy, root removed
¼ cup	water
½ cup	cooked brown rice, warm
½ cup	chopped mango
¼ cup	shredded carrots
¼ cup	sliced green onion (approx. 2 medium stalks)

Special Equipment:

Nonstick cooking spray

1. Place soy sauce, sugar, garlic powder, ground ginger, and curry powder in a microwave-safe bowl; microwave for 20 seconds on high, until sugar dissolves. Stir; set aside.

2. Sprinkle cornstarch evenly over both sides of tofu; set aside.

3. Heat a medium nonstick skillet, lightly coated with nonstick cooking spray, over medium-high heat; add sesame oil. When oil is hot, add tofu and cook for 3 to 4 minutes per side, until golden brown. Remove tofu from pan; set aside. Leave heat on.

4. To the same pan, add bok choy and water; cover and steam for 2 minutes, until tender-crisp.

5. Add brown rice to a medium serving bowl; top with bok choy, tofu, mango, and carrots. Garnish with green onion and drizzle with sauce.

Nutrition Information (per serving): Calories: 445 / Total Fat: 15 g / Saturated Fat: 2 g / Cholesterol: 0 mg / Sodium: 784 mg / Carbohydrates: 54 g / Fiber: 5 g / Sugars: 17 g / Protein: 25 g

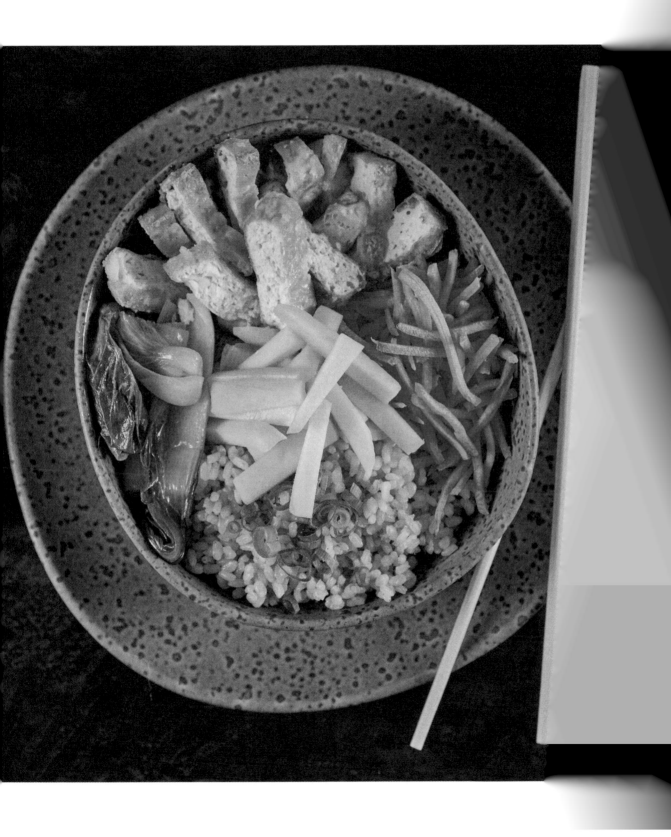

Buffalo Chicken Celery Sticks

Serves: 4 (approx. 6 sticks each)   **Prep Time:** 15 min. + 30 min. to chill   **Cooking Time:** None
Container Equivalents (per serving): ⬛1 ⬛½ ⬛½ ⬛—½

For Buffalo Sauce:

3 Tbsp.	hot pepper sauce (preferably Frank's)
2 tsp.	ghee (organic grass-fed, if possible)
2 Tbsp.	water
¼ tsp.	garlic powder
¼ tsp.	onion powder
¼ tsp.	ground smoked paprika
1 dash	sea salt (or Himalayan salt)
½ tsp.	cornstarch (preferably GMO-free) + 1 tsp. water (combine to make a slurry)

For Sticks:

1½ cups	chopped cooked chicken breast, skinless, boneless
½ cup	low-fat cream cheese
8	medium stalks celery, cut into 4-inch sticks

1. To make buffalo sauce, place a medium saucepan over medium-high heat; add hot pepper sauce, ghee, water, garlic powder, onion powder, paprika, and salt; bring to a boil, then reduce heat to a simmer.

2. Add cornstarch slurry; whisk until thickened, about 1 minute. Set sauce aside to cool, then chill in refrigerator before proceeding.

3. Add chicken, cream cheese, and chilled buffalo sauce to a food processor; pulse until pureed but slightly chunky.

4. Fill the hollow of each celery stick with 1 Tbsp. chicken mixture.

Recipe Notes:

- Serve with 2 Tbsp. *FIXATE* Ranch Dressing for dipping.

FIXATE-Approved Ranch Dressing

1 cup	reduced-fat (2%) plain yogurt
½ cup	low-fat (1%) buttermilk
2 tsp.	Dijon mustard
1 tsp.	fresh lemon juice
1 Tbsp.	chopped chives
¾ tsp.	garlic powder
¾ tsp.	onion powder
½ tsp.	sea salt (or Himalayan salt)
¼ tsp.	ground black pepper

- Combine ingredients in a medium bowl and whisk to blend.

Recipe Notes:

- Makes 12 (approx. 2 Tbsp.) servings and can be stored in an airtight container in the refrigerator for 4 to 5 days.

Nutrition Information (per serving): Calories: 187 / Total Fat: 9 g / Saturated Fat: 5 g / Cholesterol: 73 mg / Sodium: 947 mg / Carbohydrates: 7 g / Fiber: 2 g / Sugars: 3 g / Protein: 19 g

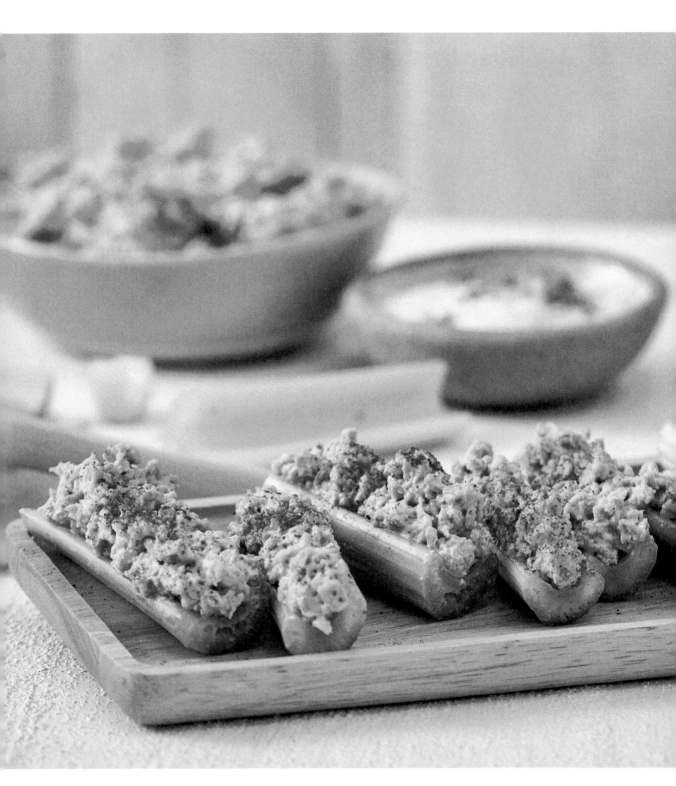

Individual 7-Layer Dip

Serves: 4 (approx. 1½ cups each) **Prep Time:** 15 min. **Cooking Time:** None
Container Equivalents (per serving): ■1 ■½ ■1 ■½

¼ cup	sour cream
½ tsp.	low-sodium taco seasoning
1 tsp.	fresh lime juice
1 cup	nonfat refried beans
½ cup	guacamole
½ cup	fresh salsa (or pico de gallo)
¼ cup	shredded cheddar jack cheese
½ cup	shredded romaine lettuce
¼ cup	sliced black olives (drained)
3 cups	carrot and celery sticks

1. In a small bowl, combine sour cream, taco seasoning, and lime juice; set aside.

2. In each of 4 small bowls or ramekins, layer ¼ cup refried beans, 2 Tbsp. guacamole, 2 Tbsp. salsa, 1 Tbsp. sour cream mixture, 1 Tbsp. cheese, 2 Tbsp. shredded lettuce, and 1 Tbsp. black olives.

3. Serve each bowl with ¾ cup carrots and celery sticks for dipping.

Nutrition Information (per serving): Calories: 212 / Total Fat: 11 g / Saturated Fat: 4 g / Cholesterol: 15 mg / Sodium: 736 mg / Carbohydrates: 24 g / Fiber: 8 g / Sugars: 6 g / Protein: 8 g

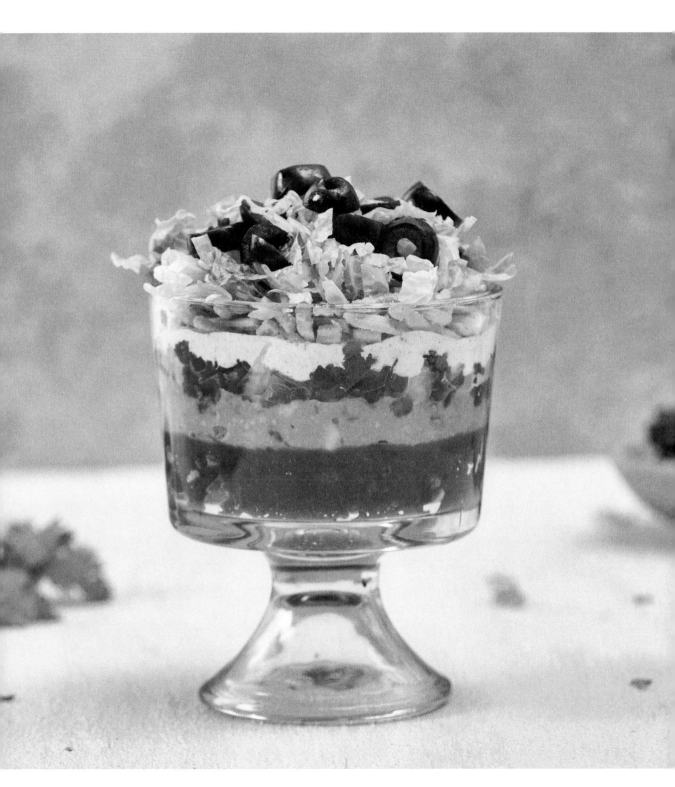

Garlic Parmesan Popcorn

Serves: 2 (approx. 2 cups each) **Prep Time:** 2 min. **Cooking Time:** 4 min.

Container Equivalents (per serving): ▢1 ■½ ●—2

1 Tbsp.+ 1 tsp.	melted ghee (organic grass-fed, if possible)
1 dash	garlic powder
4 cups	air-popped popcorn
¼ cup	grated Parmesan cheese
¼ tsp.	sea salt (or Himalayan salt)

1. Mix ghee and garlic powder in a small bowl while ghee is still hot.

2. Place popcorn in a large mixing bowl; drizzle with ghee mixture and toss to coat.

3. Add Parmesan and salt; toss again. Enjoy!

Nutrition Information (per serving): Calories: 191 / Total Fat: 13 g / Saturated Fat: 8 g / Cholesterol: 35 mg / Sodium: 477 mg / Carbohydrates: 14 g / Fiber: 2 g / Sugars: 0 g / Protein: 5 g

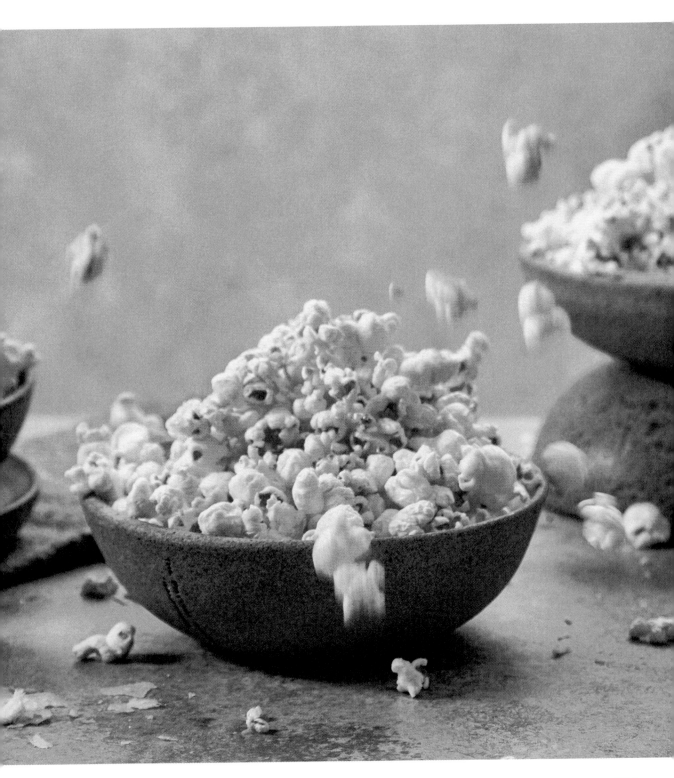

Chicken Alfredo

Serves: 4 (approx. 1 cup each) **Prep Time:** 25 min. **Cooking Time:** 5 min.
Container Equivalents (per serving): ▪️ ½ ▪️ ½ ▫️ 1½ ▪️ 1 🥄— ½

1 cup	low-fat (2%) milk
2 tsp.	unsalted organic grass-fed butter
2	cloves garlic, finely chopped
¼ tsp.	ground black pepper
2 cups	cooked whole-grain pasta
2 cups	chopped broccoli florets, steamed
1½ cups	chopped cooked chicken breast, skinless, boneless
1 cup	grated Parmesan cheese

1. Place a large skillet over medium heat. Add milk, butter, garlic, and pepper; bring to a simmer.

2. Stir in pasta, broccoli, chicken, and cheese. Continue to stir for about 2 minutes, until cheese has emulsified and a creamy sauce forms.

Recipe Note:

- To make this recipe gluten-free you can use a quinoa, brown rice, or chickpea pasta.

Nutrition Information (per serving): Calories: 356 / Total Fat: 12 g / Saturated Fat: 6 g / Cholesterol: 78 mg / Sodium: 841 mg / Carbohydrates: 33 g / Fiber: 4 g / Sugars: 4 g / Protein: 29 g

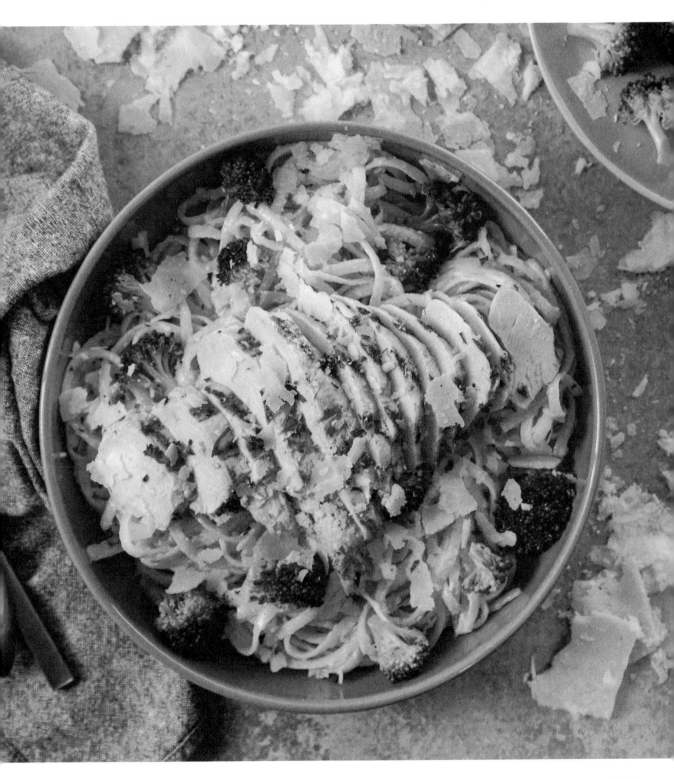

Healthy Burger Bowls

Serves: 4 (approx. 2½ cups each)   **Prep Time:** 20 min.   **Cooking Time:** 10 min.
Container Equivalents (per serving):   ■ 1½ ■ 1 ■ 1 ■ 1 ●——1

For Burger Bowl:

1 lb.	raw extra-lean ground beef
¼ tsp.	sea salt (or Himalayan salt)
¼ tsp.	ground black pepper
1 cup	sliced onion (approx. 1 medium)
3 cups	chopped romaine lettuce
1 cup	halved grape tomatoes
1 cup	sliced dill pickles
8 slices	cooked turkey bacon, chopped
1 cup	shredded cheddar cheese

For Special Sauce:

3 Tbsp.	mayonnaise (preferably olive oil–based)
2 Tbsp.	all-natural ketchup
2 tsp.	pickle relish
1 tsp.	finely chopped onion
1 pinch	sea salt (or Himalayan salt)

Special Equipment:

Nonstick cooking spray

1. Heat a large skillet, lightly coated with spray, over high heat until very hot.

2. Add ground beef, salt, and pepper and cook, stirring to separate meat into crumbles, about 5 minutes, until browned and cooked through.

3. Remove ground beef from pan with a slotted spoon; transfer to a plate lined with paper towels. Leave heat on.

4. Add onions to pan and cook without stirring for 2 to 3 minutes; flip and cook for 2 to 3 minutes more until browned on both sides.

5. To make special sauce, combine mayonnaise, ketchup, pickle relish, chopped onion, and salt in a small bowl.

6. To assemble burger bowls, evenly divide lettuce among 4 bowls (approx. ¾ cup each). Top evenly with ¼ cup tomatoes, ¼ cup pickles, ¼ cup cooked onion, a quarter of the bacon (approx. 2 slices), and ¼ cup cheese. Drizzle evenly with special sauce (approx. 1 Tbsp. + 1½ tsp. each).

Nutrition Information (per serving): Calories: 447 / Total Fat: 28 g / Saturated Fat: 10 g / Cholesterol: 130 mg / Sodium: 1,353 mg / Carbohydrates: 14 g / Fiber: 2 g / Sugars: 7 g / Protein: 38 g

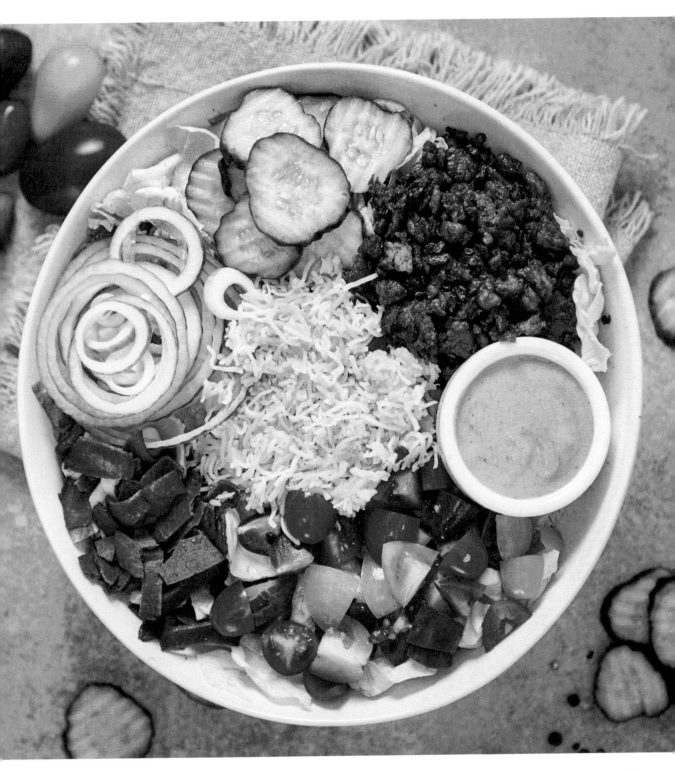

Slow-Cooker Asian Chicken

Serves: 4 (approx. 1¼ cups each) **Prep Time:** 12 min. **Cooking Time:** 4 to 5 hrs.
Container Equivalents (per serving): ⬛ ½ ⬛ 1 ⬜ 1½ ⬛ ½

4 oz.	dry linguini
1 lb.	raw chicken breast, skinless, boneless
1 cup	sliced red bell pepper
½ cup	shredded carrot (approx. 1 medium)
½ cup	chopped onion (approx. ⅔ medium)
2	cloves garlic, finely chopped
1 cup	low-sodium organic chicken broth
3 Tbsp.	reduced-sodium tamari soy sauce
1 Tbsp.	all-natural peanut butter
1 Tbsp.	coconut sugar
¼ cup	chopped fresh cilantro
1 Tbsp.	fresh lime juice
28	peanuts (roasted, unsalted), coarsely chopped

1. Bring a small pot of water to a boil over high heat. Add linguini and cook for 2 to 3 minutes, until flexible; drain.

2. Add linguini, chicken, bell pepper, carrot, onion, garlic, chicken broth, soy sauce, peanut butter, and coconut sugar to a slow cooker; stir to combine. Cover and cook on low for 4 to 5 hours, until chicken falls apart easily.

3. Shred chicken with 2 forks.

4. Divide chicken evenly among 4 plates; top evenly with cilantro, lime juice, and chopped peanuts.

Nutrition Information (per serving): Calories: 360 / Total Fat: 9 g / Saturated Fat: 2 g / Cholesterol: 84 mg / Sodium: 614 mg / Carbohydrates: 32 g / Fiber: 3 g / Sugars: 6 g / Protein: 35 g

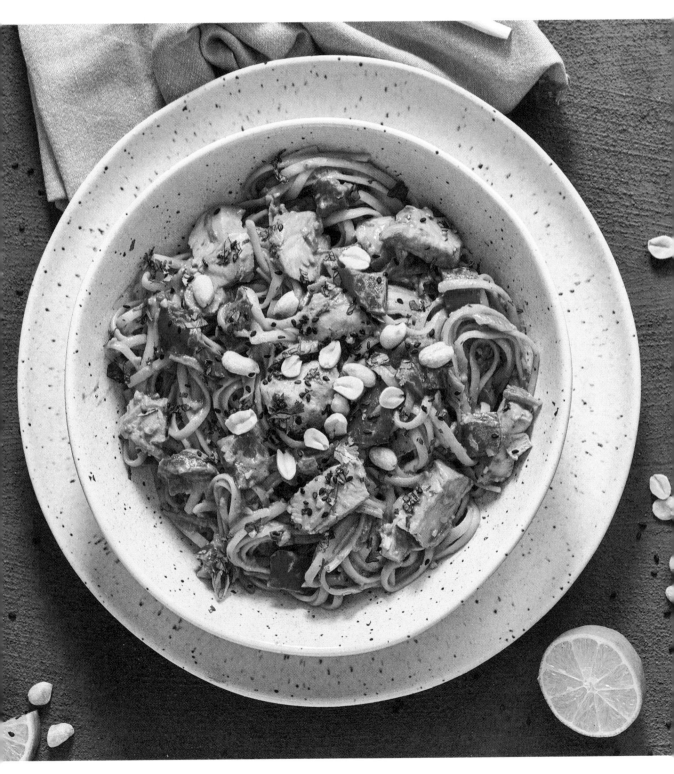

Steak Chimichurri

Serves: 4 (4-oz. portions steak, approx. 2 Tbsp. chimichurri)
Prep Time: 10 min.　**Cooking Time:** 10 min.
Container Equivalents (per serving): 　■ 1　■ 1　●— 1

For Chimichurri:

3 Tbsp.	extra-virgin olive oil
2 Tbsp.	sherry vinegar
1 tsp.	coconut sugar
¼ tsp.	sea salt (or Himalayan salt)
¼ tsp.	ground black pepper
1 clove	garlic, finely chopped
2 Tbsp.	finely chopped fresh parsley
2 Tbsp.	finely chopped fresh cilantro
1 Tbsp.	finely chopped fresh oregano
1 tsp.	finely chopped, seeded Fresno or other hot chili (optional)

For Steak:

1 lb.	raw skirt or flank steak
1 dash	sea salt (or Himalayan salt)
1 dash	ground black pepper
1 tsp.	ghee (organic grass-fed, if possible), melted

1. To make chimichurri, combine olive oil, vinegar, sugar, salt, pepper, garlic, parsley, cilantro, oregano, and Fresno chili in a small mixing bowl; stir to combine. Set aside.

2. Preheat a large skillet over high heat.

3. Season steak on both sides with salt and pepper; rub all over with ghee.

4. When pan is very hot, add steak and cook 3 minutes per side for medium-rare, 4 minutes per side for medium. Remove from pan.

5. Rest steak 5 minutes. Thinly slice across the grain.

6. Divide steak evenly among 4 plates; top each portion with 2 Tbsp. chimichurri.

Recipe Note:
- Apple cider vinegar can be substituted for sherry vinegar.

Nutrition Information (per serving): Calories: 273 / Total Fat: 17 g / Saturated Fat: 4 g / Cholesterol: 71 mg / Sodium: 255 mg / Carbohydrates: 3 g / Fiber: 0 g / Sugars: 1 g / Protein: 25 g

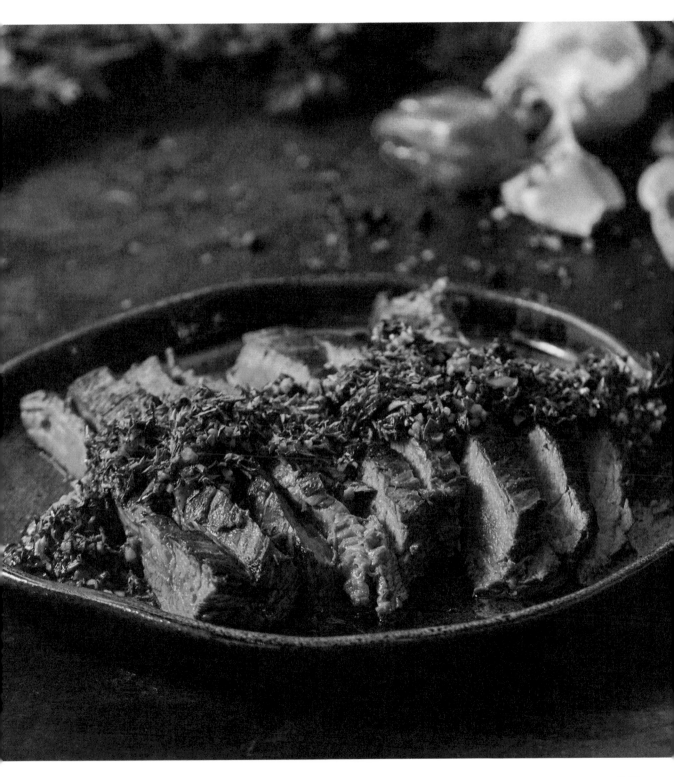

Vegan Tacos with Aji Verde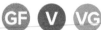

Serves: 4 (2 tacos each) **Prep Time:** 12 min. **Cooking Time:** 13 min.
Container Equivalents (per serving): 1½ ■ ½ ■ 1 ● 1
Vegan Container Equivalents (per serving): ■ 1½ ■ ½ **B** 1 ● 1

1 Tbsp.	extra-virgin olive oil
2 cups	sliced mushrooms (approx. 6 oz.)
1½ cups	crumbled organic firm tofu (approx. 7 oz.)
1 cup	chopped tomatoes (approx. 1½ medium)
½ cup	chopped onion (approx. ⅔ medium)
2	cloves garlic, finely chopped
2 tsp.	chili powder
1 tsp.	ground cumin
½ tsp.	sea salt (or Himalayan salt)
8	(6-inch) corn tortillas
1 cup	shredded cabbage
½ cup	fresh salsa (or pico de gallo)

1. Place olive oil to a large skillet over high heat until it begins to smoke. Add mushrooms and tofu and cook, stirring occasionally, for 5 minutes, until mushrooms and tofu brown.

2. Reduce heat to medium, add tomatoes, onion, garlic, chili powder, cumin, and salt. Cook for 5 to 7 minutes until tomato has broken down into a thick sauce.

3. Warm tortillas on each side in a hot, dry pan and divide evenly among 4 plates. Fill tortillas evenly with mushroom mixture (about ¼ cup each); top each taco with 2 Tbsp. cabbage and 1 Tbsp. salsa.

Serving Suggestion:

- In addition to cabbage and salsa, top each taco with 1 Tbsp. Aji Verde Sauce (see separate recipe for Aji Verde Sauce). Remember to track the ½ ■ container.

Nutritional Information (per serving): Calories: 265 / Total Fat: 9 g / Saturated Fat: 1 g / Cholesterol: 0 mg / Sodium: 484 mg / Carbohydrates: 34 g / Fiber: 6 g / Sugars: 4 g / Protein: 15 g

Aji Verde Sauce

Serves: 12 (2 Tbsp. each) **Prep Time:** 10 min. **Cooking Time:** None
Container Equivalents (per serving): ■ ½ / **Vegan Container Equivalents** (per serving): ■ ½

1 cup	cashews (soaked in water overnight)	2	cloves garlic
		½ cup	water
1 cup	fresh cilantro, leaves and tender stems	3 Tbsp.	fresh lime juice
		½ tsp.	sugar
1	medium jalapeño pepper, seeds and veins removed	½ tsp.	sea salt (or Himalayan salt)

- Place cashews, cilantro, jalapeño, garlic, water, lime juice, sugar, and salt in a blender; cover. Blend until smooth.

Recipe Notes:

- Pre-soaking the cashews overnight allows for a smoother sauce when blending.
- Store leftover sauce in an airtight container in the refrigerator for up to 5 days.

Nutrition Information (per serving): Calories: 56 / Total Fat: 4 g / Saturated Fat: 1 g / Cholesterol: 0 mg / Sodium: 101 mg / Carbohydrates: 3 g / Fiber: 0 g / Sugars: 1 g / Protein: 2 g

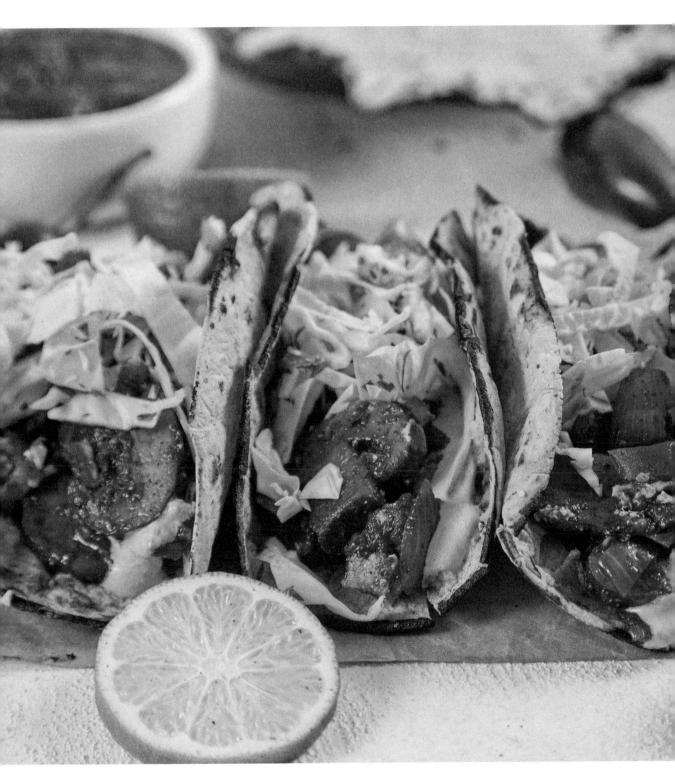

Mediterranean Spiced Carrots (GF) (VG)

Serves: 4 (approx. 1 cup each)   **Prep Time:** 10 min.   **Cooking Time:** 40 min.

Container Equivalents (per serving): ■ 1 ■ ½ ●— 2½

4 cups	baby carrots, peeled
3 Tbsp.	extra-virgin olive oil
2 Tbsp.	fresh lemon juice
3	cloves garlic, finely chopped
1 Tbsp.	finely chopped fresh ginger (or 1 tsp. ground ginger)
1 tsp.	ground cumin
1 tsp.	ground coriander
½ tsp.	ground cinnamon
½ tsp.	sea salt (or Himalayan salt)
½ tsp.	ground black pepper
½ tsp.	crushed red pepper flakes (optional)
¼ tsp.	ground cloves
½ cup	sliced almonds
¾ cup	*FIXATE* Tzatziki Sauce

1. Preheat oven to 375°F.
2. Line large baking sheet with parchment paper. Set aside.
3. Combine carrots, olive oil, lemon juice, garlic, ginger, cumin, coriander, cinnamon, salt, black pepper, crushed red pepper, and cloves in large mixing bowl; toss to combine.
4. Spread evenly on prepared baking sheet. Bake for 10 minutes.
5. Turn carrots and top with almonds; cook 25 to 30 minutes more, stirring occasionally, until tender-crisp.
6. Divide evenly among 4 plates; serve each with 3 Tbsp. *FIXATE* Tzatziki Sauce for dipping.

Recipe Notes:

- If you don't have sliced almonds, you can chop 12 raw almonds.
- You can make this recipe vegan by omitting the tzatziki sauce.

FIXATE Tzatziki Sauce

1 cup	reduced-fat (2%) plain Greek yogurt
1 Tbsp.	fresh lemon juice
1 tsp.	finely grated lemon peel (lemon zest)
1	clove garlic
½ tsp.	sea salt (or Himalayan salt)
½ cup	coarsely chopped seeded cucumber
2 tsp.	fresh dill
2 tsp.	fresh mint leaves
¼ tsp.	ground black pepper

- Combine ingredients in a food processor; process until smooth.

Recipe Notes:

- It makes 8 (approx. 3 Tbsp. each) servings and can be stored in an airtight container for up to 4 or 5 days.

Nutrition Information (per serving): Calories: 220 / Total Fat: 16 g / Saturated Fat: 2 g / Cholesterol: 0 mg / Sodium: 386 mg / Carbohydrates: 17 g / Fiber: 6 g / Sugars: 7 g / Protein: 4 g

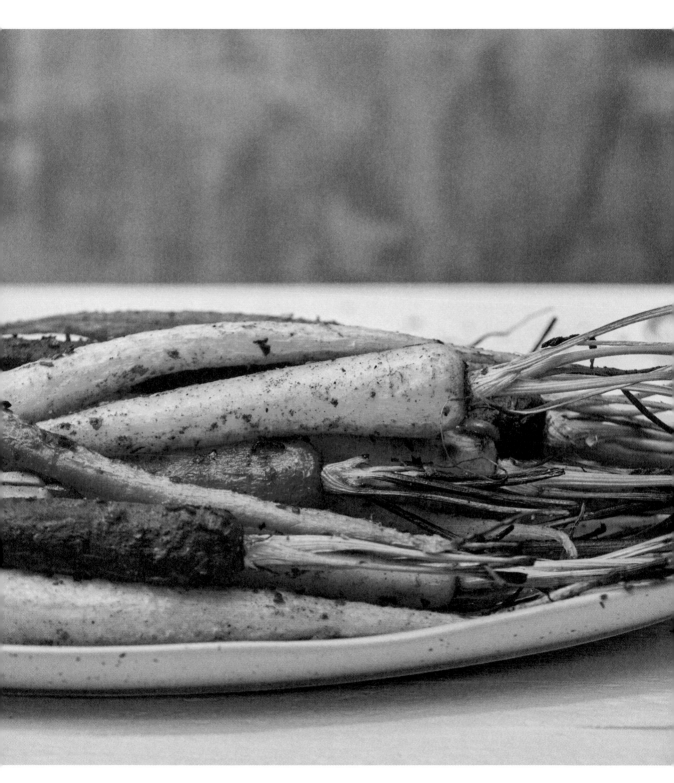

Roasted Balsamic Rosemary Mushrooms

Serves: 4 (approx. ½ cup each)   **Prep Time:** 10 min.   **Cooking Time:** 20 min.

Container Equivalents (per serving): 🟩 1 🥄 1

Vegan Container Equivalents (per serving): 🟩 1 🥄 1

3 cups	halved large mixed mushrooms
1 cup	halved grape tomatoes
2	cloves garlic, thinly sliced
1 Tbsp.	finely chopped fresh rosemary
1 Tbsp.	extra-virgin olive oil
1 Tbsp.	balsamic vinegar
¼ tsp.	sea salt (or Himalayan salt)
¼ tsp.	ground black pepper

1. Preheat oven to 425°F.

2. Place mushrooms, tomatoes, garlic, rosemary, olive oil, vinegar, salt, and pepper in a large mixing bowl; toss until well coated.

3. Arrange ingredients in a single layer in a roasting pan or casserole dish.

4. Bake for 15 to 20 minutes, until mushrooms are tender and lightly crisped around the edges.

Recipe Note:

- A rimmed baking sheet can be used if you do not have a roasting pan or casserole dish.

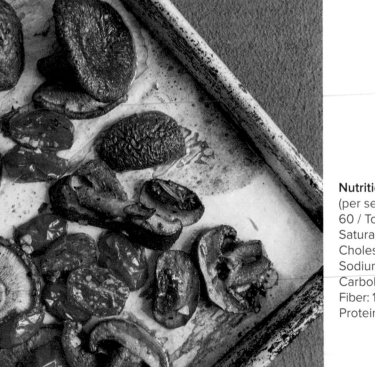

Nutrition Information
(per serving): Calories: 60 / Total Fat: 4 g / Saturated Fat: 1 g / Cholesterol: 0 mg / Sodium: 160 mg / Carbohydrates: 7 g / Fiber: 1 g / Sugars: 3 g / Protein: 3 g

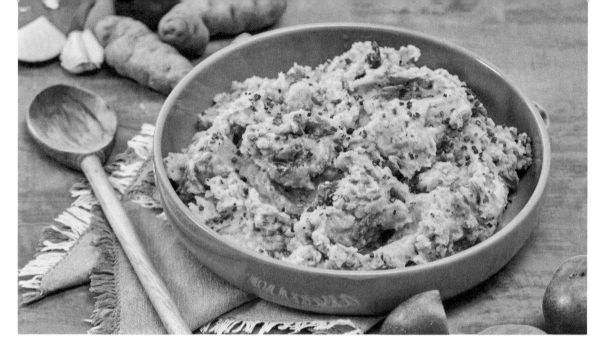

Roast Garlic Mashed Potatoes

Serves: 4 (approx. ½ cup each)   **Prep Time:** 15 min.   **Cooking Time:** 1 hr. 15 min.

Container Equivalents (per serving): ▢ 1 ●— ½

1	bulb garlic
2 cups	chopped russet potatoes (skin on, washed)
1 Tbsp.	ghee (organic grass-fed, if possible)
4	fresh sage leaves
3 Tbsp.	unsweetened almond milk, warm
¼ tsp. + 1 dash	sea salt (or Himalayan salt)
¼ tsp.	ground black pepper

Special Equipment:

Olive oil cooking spray

Aluminum foil

1. Preheat oven to 350°F.

2. Cut off top quarter of garlic bulb, exposing inner cloves. Spray lightly with olive oil cooking spray and wrap in aluminum foil; bake for 1 hour, or until garlic cloves are golden brown. Set aside to cool slightly.

3. Place potatoes in a medium pot and cover with water. Place pot over high heat and cook for 10 to 15 minutes, or until soft.

4. While potatoes cook, melt ghee in a small pan over medium heat. Add sage leaves and cook for 2 to 4 minutes, until crisp. Remove from heat; set aside.

5. Drain potatoes and place in a large mixing bowl; add ghee mixture, almond milk, salt, and pepper.

6. Squeeze garlic bulb to release inner cloves, being careful to pick out any loose skins; add garlic to bowl.

7. Mash all ingredients together with a potato masher or the back of a fork.

Nutrition Information (per serving): Calories: 91 / Total Fat: 4 g / Saturated Fat: 2 g / Cholesterol: 10 mg / Sodium: 180 mg / Carbohydrates: 14 g / Fiber: 1 g / Sugars: 1 g / Protein: 2 g

Blondies

Serves: 12 (1 blondie each) **Prep Time:** 13 min. **Cooking Time:** 17 min.
Container Equivalents (per serving): ▪ ½ ▪ 1 ▪— 1

1 cup	almond flour
¼ tsp.	sea salt (or Himalayan salt)
½ tsp.	baking powder, gluten-free
¼ cup	butter, melted
½ cup	light brown sugar
1	large egg
1 tsp.	pure vanilla extract
¼ cup	white chocolate chips

Special equipment:

Baking pan

Parchment paper

1. Preheat oven to 350°F.

2. Line 8-in. x 8-in. baking pan with parchment paper, leaving extra to come up the sides of the pan (this will help you lift out finished blondies). Set aside.

3. Place almond flour, salt, and baking powder in a medium mixing bowl; whisk to combine.

4. Place butter, brown sugar, egg, and vanilla in another mixing bowl; whisk to combine.

5. Add flour mixture to ghee mixture; whisk until well combined. Fold in white chocolate chips.

6. Pour batter into prepared baking pan and bake 14 to 17 minutes, until just beginning to brown.

7. Let cool completely; cut into 12 pieces.

Nutrition Information (per serving): Calories: 161 / Total Fat: 11 g / Saturated Fat: 5 g / Cholesterol: 31 mg / Sodium: 62 mg / Carbohydrates: 14 g / Fiber: 1 g / Sugars: 12 g / Protein: 3 g

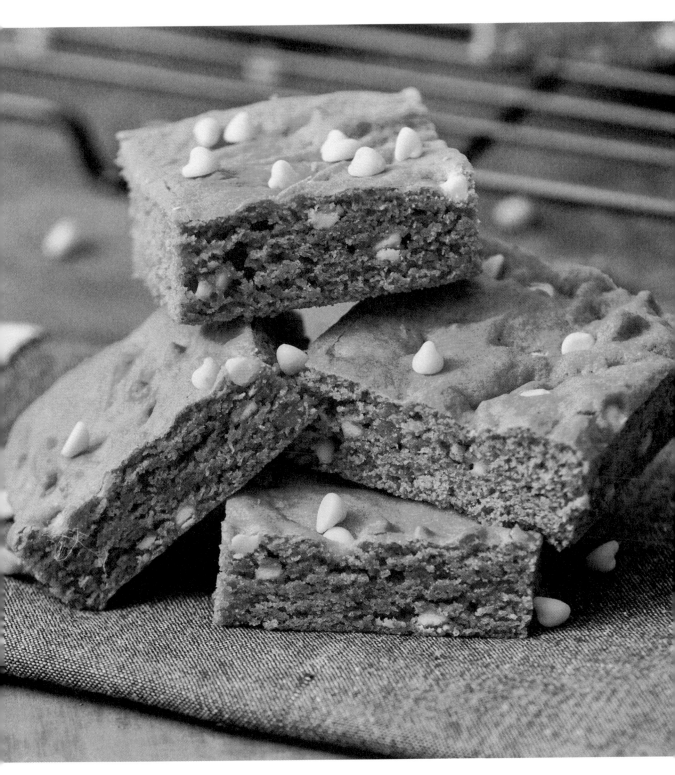

Lemon Meringue Pies

Serves: 12 (1 mini pie each) **Prep Time:** 43 min. + 45 min. to chill **Cooking Time:** 17 min.

Container Equivalents (per serving): ⬜ 1½ ⬛ ½ ⬤— 2

For Crust:

2½ cups crushed gluten-free graham crackers

¼ cup + 3 Tbsp. extra-virgin organic coconut oil

1 Tbsp. pure maple syrup

For Lemon Filling:

1 cup fresh lemon juice

1 cup canned coconut cream, well shaken

½ cup pure maple syrup

1 dash sea salt (or Himalayan salt)

3 Tbsp. cornstarch (preferably GMO-free) + 3 Tbsp. water (combine to make a slurry)

1 Tbsp. finely grated lemon peel (lemon zest)

For Meringue:

2 Tbsp. + 2 tsp. water

2 tsp. cornstarch (preferably GMO-free)

3 large egg whites (approx. ⅓ cup)

¼ tsp. pure vanilla extract

1 dash cream of tartar

3 Tbsp. pure maple syrup

1. Preheat oven to 325°F.

2. Prepare twelve muffin cups by lining with muffin papers; coat lightly with nonstick cooking spray. Set aside.

3. To make crust, place graham crackers in a food processor or blender; pulse until fine. Add coconut oil and maple syrup; pulse until thoroughly combined.

4. Divide crust mixture evenly among muffin cups (approx. 3 Tbsp. each) and press down with fingers, molding it onto the bottom and sides of each cup. Place in freezer to set.

5. To make lemon filling, place a medium saucepan over high heat. Add lemon juice, coconut cream, maple syrup, and salt. Bring to a boil, then reduce to a simmer.

6. Whisk in cornstarch slurry; cook for 1 minute, until sauce thickens. Remove from heat; stir in lemon peel.

7. Pour lemon filling into a medium bowl; place bowl in an ice bath until lukewarm.

8. To make meringue, place a small saucepan over medium heat. Add water and cornstarch, whisking constantly until a thick gel forms; set aside.

9. Place egg whites, vanilla, and cream of tartar in a large mixing bowl; beat with a hand mixer until frothy. Slowly add maple syrup, beating constantly, until soft peaks form.

10. Continue to beat egg white mixture while adding the cornstarch mixture, a little bit at a time, until stiff peaks form.

11. Divide lemon filling evenly among muffin cups (approx. ¼ cup each); top evenly with meringue (approx. ¼ cup each). Bake for 14 to 17 minutes, until meringue is golden brown.

12. Chill in refrigerator until lemon mixture has set before serving.

Nutrition Information (per serving): Calories: 265 / Total Fat: 14 g / Saturated Fat: 11 g / Cholesterol: 0 mg / Sodium: 132 mg / Carbohydrates: 34 g / Fiber: 0 g / Sugars: 19 g / Protein: 3 g

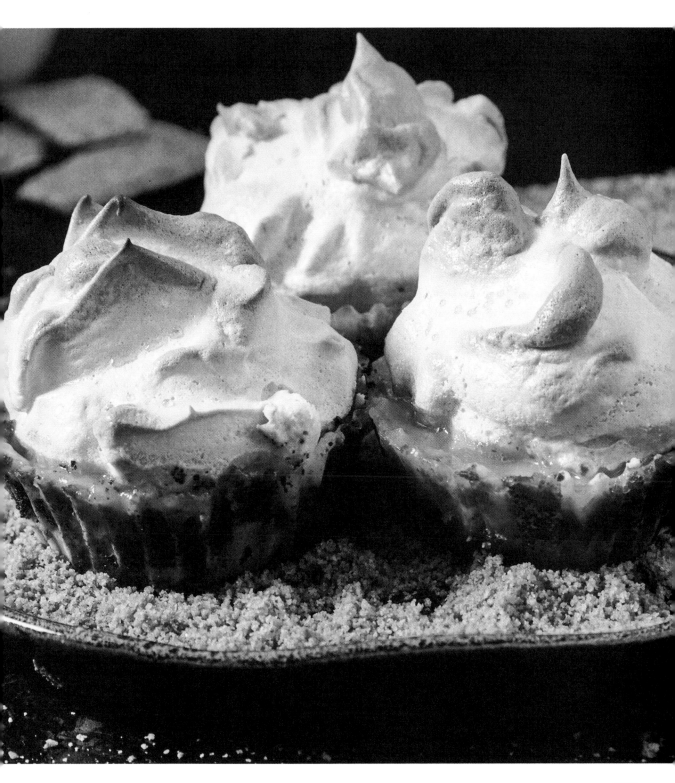

Peanut Butter Apple Pie Cookies

Serves: 10 (1 cookie each)   **Prep Time:** 14 min.   **Cooking Time:** 11 min.
Container Equivalents (per serving):   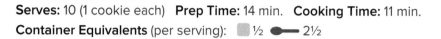 ½ 🥄 2½

½ cup	dry rolled oats, gluten-free
½ cup	almond flour
3 Tbsp.	coconut sugar
1 tsp.	baking soda, gluten-free
¼ tsp.	sea salt (or Himalayan salt)
¼ tsp.	ground cinnamon
¼ tsp.	ground nutmeg
1 dash	ground cardamom
1	large egg
½ cup	all-natural peanut butter
¼ cup	all-natural, unsweetened applesauce
1 tsp.	fresh lemon juice

1. Preheat oven to 350°F.

2. Line large baking sheet with parchment paper and lightly coat with nonstick cooking spray. Set aside.

3. Place oats, almond flour, coconut sugar, baking soda, salt, cinnamon, nutmeg, and cardamom in a food processor. Pulse until oats are finely ground.

4. Add egg, peanut butter, applesauce, and lemon juice. Process until a sticky dough forms.

5. Drop by rounding 2 Tbsp. onto prepared baking sheet, to form 10 cookies; leave 1 inch of space between each cookie.

6. Bake for 9 to 11 minutes, until just beginning to brown around edges. Cool completely before serving.

Recipe Note:

- You can substitute other nut butters for peanut butter.

Special Equipment:

Baking sheet

Parchment paper

Nonstick cooking spray

Nutrition Information (per serving): Calories: 152 / Total Fat: 10 g / Saturated Fat: 1 g / Cholesterol: 22 mg / Sodium: 69 mg / Carbohydrates: 10 g / Fiber: 2 g / Sugars: 4 g / Protein: 5 g

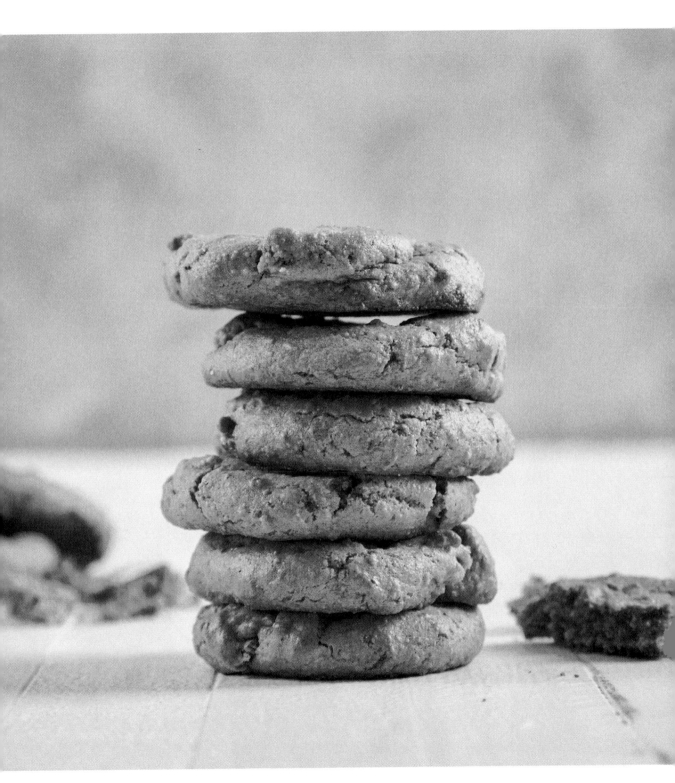

Vegan Chocolate Chip Scones (GF) (V) (VG)

Serves: 10 (1 scone each) **Prep Time:** 35 min. + 1 hr. **Cooking Time:** 18 min.

Container Equivalents (per serving): ▢ 1½ ▬● 1½

Vegan Container Equivalents (per serving): Ⓑ 1½ ▬● 1½

2 cups	gluten-free all-purpose flour (preferably Bob's Red Mill All-Purpose Baking Flour, red label)	1. Place flour, coconut sugar, baking powder, and salt in a food processor; pulse to combine.
¼ cup	coconut sugar	2. Add coconut oil; pulse until evenly mixed.
1¼ tsp.	baking powder, gluten-free	3. Add coconut milk and vanilla; pulse until dough forms.
¼ tsp.	sea salt (or Himalayan salt)	4. Turn dough out onto a clean surface; knead in chocolate chips. Wrap with plastic wrap and use hands to flatten into a ½-inch-thick disk. Refrigerate for 1 hour.
¼ cup	extra-virgin organic coconut oil, solid	5. Preheat oven to 350°F; line a large baking sheet with parchment paper.
½ cup	canned light coconut milk	6. Divide dough into 10 equal pieces (re-form scrap ends into a whole if necessary). Arrange on prepared baking sheet; sprinkle evenly with sugar.
1 tsp.	pure vanilla extract	7. Bake for 15 to 18 minutes, until lightly browned and a toothpick inserted into the center comes out clean.
¼ cup	semisweet mini chocolate chips, dairy-free	
1 tsp.	organic raw sugar	

Special Equipment:

Plastic wrap

Baking sheet

Parchment paper

Nutrition Information (per serving): Calories: 198 / Total Fat: 7 g / Saturated Fat: 6 g / Cholesterol: 0 mg / Sodium: 73 mg / Carbohydrates: 31 g / Fiber: 1 g / Sugars: 6 g / Protein: 2 g

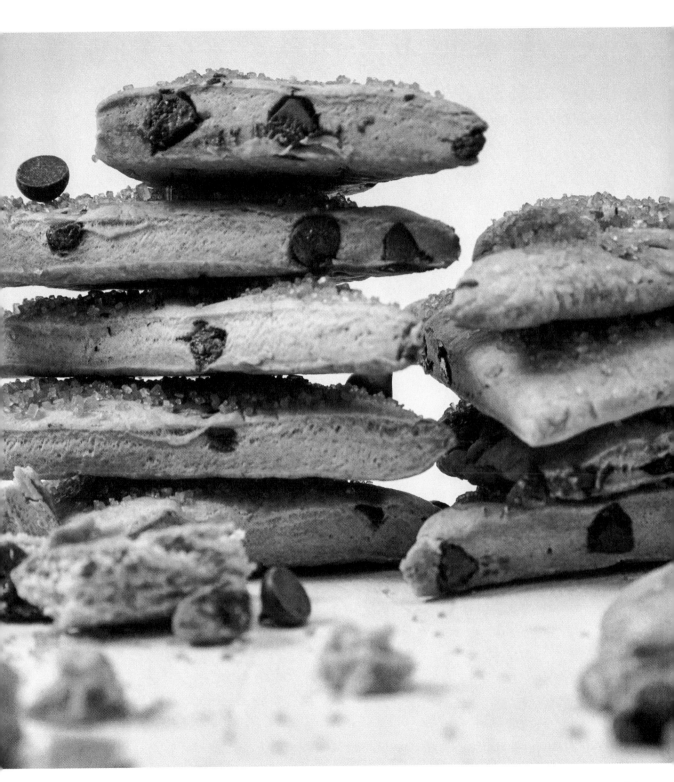

Pomegranate Margarita

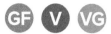

Serves: 1 (approx. 5 fl. oz.) **Prep Time:** 5 min.

Container Equivalents (per serving): ▪ ½ ▫ 1

Vegan Container Equivalents (per serving): ▪ ½ **B** 1

	Ice
1 fl. oz.	tequila
2 fl. oz.	pomegranate juice
1 fl. oz.	fresh lime juice
¼ fl. oz.	Cointreau or Triple Sec
1	lime wedge
1 tsp.	fresh pomegranate seeds

1. Fill a rocks glass three-quarters full with ice.
2. Add tequila, pomegranate juice, lime juice, and Cointreau or Triple Sec.
3. Stir to chill; garnish with lime wedge and pomegranate seeds.

Recipe Note:

- The rocks glass (or old-fashioned glass) is a short tumbler used for serving spirits, such as whiskey, with ice cubes.

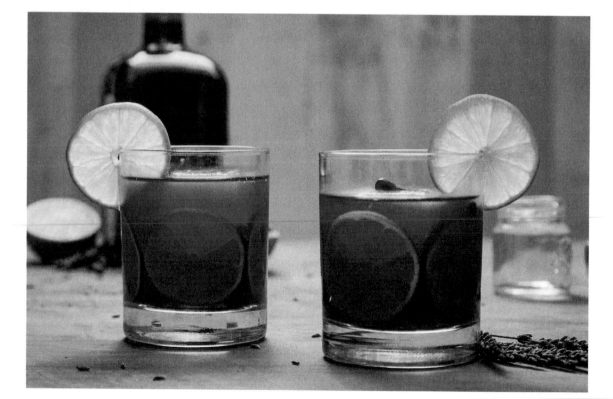

Nutrition Information (per serving): Calories: 136 / Total Fat: 1 g / Saturated Fat: 0 g / Cholesterol: 0 mg / Sodium: 3 mg / Carbohydrates: 14 g / Fiber: 2 g / Sugars: 10 g / Protein: 1 g

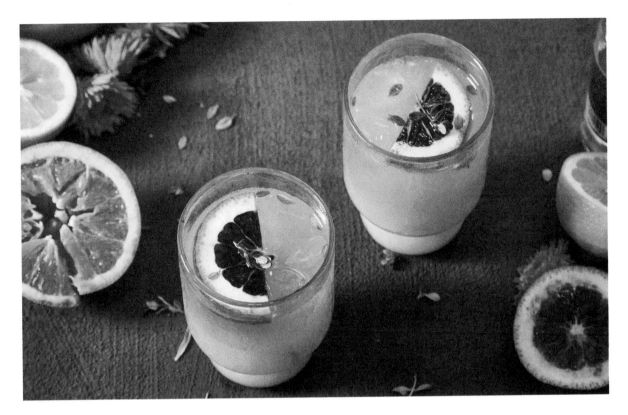

Sunset Frizzante

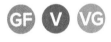

Serves: 1 (approx. 5½ fl. oz.)   **Prep Time:** 5 min.
Container Equivalents (per serving): ■ ½ ▨ 1
Vegan Container Equivalents (per serving): ■ ½ **B** 1

	Ice
1 fl. oz.	vodka
½ fl. oz.	Campari
2 fl. oz.	fresh orange juice
1 tsp.	fresh lemon juice
2 fl. oz.	club soda
1 slice	orange

1. Fill a wineglass three-quarters full with ice.
2. Add vodka, Campari, orange juice, and lemon juice; mix well.
3. Top with club soda; garnish with orange.

Recipe Note:

- Campari is an Italian aperitif with a bitter, spicy, and sweet flavor.

Nutrition Information (per serving): Calories: 134 / Total Fat: 0 g / Saturated Fat: 0 g / Cholesterol: 0 mg / Sodium: 13 mg / Carbohydrates: 11 g / Fiber: 0 g / Sugars: 5 g / Protein: 0 g

GET FIT, STRONG & HEALTHY

The goal of this book is to lose weight like crazy. A huge part of that happens through nutrition, what you put into your body. But the other piece of the puzzle is exercise. I'm a huge proponent of exercise. Exercise has tremendous health benefits: It strengthens your muscles, heart, and lungs, it can help increase bone mass and reduce stress; building lean muscle helps burn more calories hours after you've stopped exercising, and all the toning and tightening helps you look and feel even better in your own skin.

On the following pages, I've created 2 fast-paced, effective 30-minute workouts that you can do just about anywhere. The first is a cardio workout that requires nothing but you. The second is a total-body sculpting workout to get you moving that requires nothing more than a set of hand weights.

I encourage you to visit TeamACWorkouts.com to follow along with me at home.

WORKOUT #1
CARDIO FIX 2.0

Get your heart pumping and your body moving as you melt away the pounds with this fast-paced 30-minute routine.

How It Works: Before you begin, do a 3-minute warm-up to get your heart rate up and the blood flowing to muscles to prevent injury. DON'T skip it!

Cardio Fix 2.0 is eight moves and one bonus move. You will do each move for 60 seconds. You know what I say . . . You can do anything for 60 seconds! After completing one exercise, rest for 30 seconds. Then move to the next exercise for 60 seconds. Rest for 30 seconds and repeat the 2-move sequence once more before moving on to the next pair of exercises. At the end of all 4 rounds, perform the bonus move twice, for 60 seconds each time, with a 30-second break in between. Finish with a 3-minute cooldown.

Equipment Needed: water, towel

WORKOUT #2
DIRTY 30 SCULPT

Build strength and burn calories with this quick 30-minute strength workout.

How It Works: Before you begin the workout, do a 3-minute warm-up to get your heart rate up and the blood flowing to your muscles to prevent injury. This is really important. DON'T skip it. I've recommended some good warm-up moves on the following pages.

Dirty 30 Sculpt is made up of 8 exercises. You will do each move for 60 seconds. Rest for 30 seconds between exercises. After completing the second exercise in each pair, repeat the 2-move sequence once. After the workout, do a 3-minute cooldown.

Equipment Needed: water, light and/or medium dumbbells

Safety Note: Consult your physician and follow all safety instructions before beginning any exercise program, especially if you are pregnant, breastfeeding, have any medical condition, or are taking any medication.

CARDIO FIX 2.0

Warm-Up (3 minutes)

(Don't Skip This!)
Perform each warm-up move for 15 seconds. After completing the 6 moves, without resting, do a second round at a faster pace.

- **High Knees:** March in place, raising your knees as high as you can.

- **Jog in Place:** Bring your heels up toward your booty.

- **Jumping Jacks:** Do standard jumping jacks, just like in grade school.

- **Windmills:** With abs in and chest up, make wide circles with your straight arms. Halfway through, reverse the circle.

- **Over-the-Top Side Stretch:** With feet shoulder-width apart, raise your right arm toward the ceiling and do a side bend to the left. Reverse with the left arm to the right.

- **Alternating Toe Touch:** With feet shoulder-width apart, form a T with your torso by holding your arms out to your sides, parallel with the floor. Now swing your right arm down and bend at the waist to touch your right hand to your left toes. Return to start and repeat with your left hand to right toes.

Cardio Moves

Perform the moves in pairs (or "supersets"), doing each for 60 seconds and resting 30 seconds between them. Do each superset twice. Finish with the bonus move twice for 60 seconds followed by the cooldown.

1. Sumo Jack
2. Heel Tap Hop

3. Lateral Toe Tap
4. Plank Toe Tap

5. Front Curtsy Lunge
6. Burpee Jack

7. Cross-Country Skier to Ex Jump
8. Two Side Shuffle to One Half-Skater

Bonus Move: Knee Pull, Up/Down, Hip Drop

Cooldown (3 minutes)

- Inhale, raising arms overhead; exhale lowering arms. Repeat.

- **Hamstring stretch:** While standing, roll forward, reaching for your toes. Hold the stretch for 10 seconds, then roll back up. Repeat.

- **Quad stretch:** Hold onto something for balance. Bend your right knee and grab your toes on your right foot, pulling your heel up to your butt. Keep your knees close together and press your pelvis forward slightly. Hold for 10 seconds, then repeat with the other leg.

- **Shoulder stretch:** Take your right arm straight across your chest. Grab your right wrist with your left hand, and pull that arm toward you. Press your right shoulder down. Hold 10 seconds and repeat with the left arm.

Sumo Jack

1. Start with feet close together, heels nearly touching, and arms raised straight above your head.

2. When you jump your feet out like a regular jumping jack, swing your arms down in front of you and land your feet wide, toes pointing outward.

3. Bend your knees to lower into a mini sumo or half sumo.

4. Next, jump your feet together and swing your arms above you again. Repeat. Stay light on your toes. Your knees will track over the toes. Keep your abs in.

Heel Tap Hop

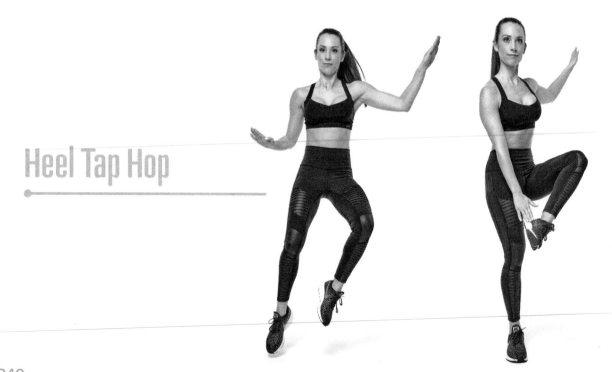

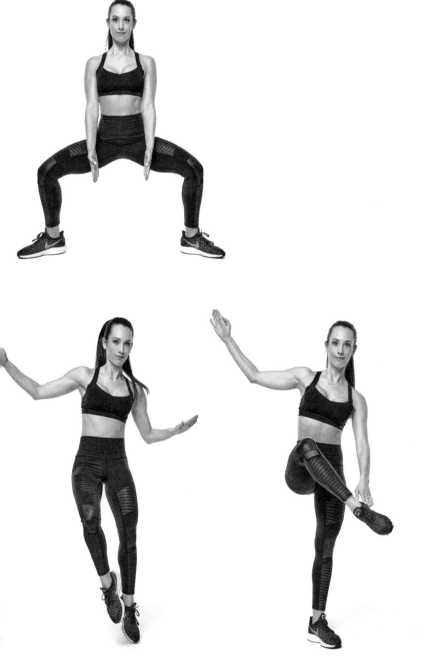

1. Start with your feet hip-width apart and jump side to side, bringing one heel at a time toward your opposite knee and tapping that heel with your hand—right hand to left heel, left hand to right heel.

2. If that's too difficult, a modification would be to not hop, but just lift up each heel to tap it with the opposite hand and alternate right hand to left heel, left hand to right heel.

Lateral Toe Tap

1. Stand with feet hip-width apart.

2. Keeping your core engaged, chest up, and back flat, hop your right foot out to your side as you push your hips back, lower your body, and touch the floor inside your left foot with your right hand.

3. Switch legs, bringing your right leg in, hopping your left leg out to your side, and touching the floor on the inside of your right foot with your left hand.

4. Continue alternating sides with each rep.

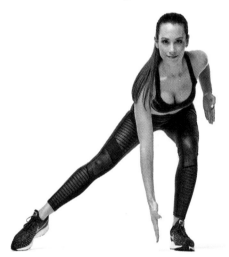

Plank Toe Tap

1. Assume a high plank position with your hands on the floor directly under your shoulders, your feet hip-width apart, and head aligned with your spine so your back forms a straight line from your head to your heels.

2. Draw your bellybutton in. Now, press back, shifting your hips up toward the ceiling and reaching your right hand back toward your left toes, which remain on the floor.

3. Return to the starting position. Next, press back, lift your hips toward the ceiling and reach with your left hand toward your right toes. Repeat.

4. Continue alternating sides with each rep.

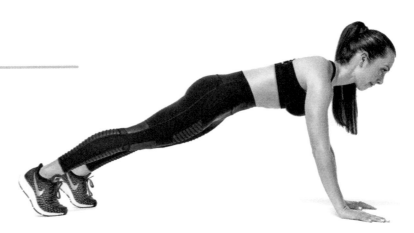

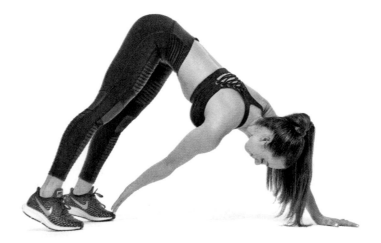

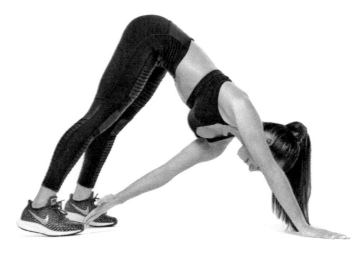

Front Curtsy Lunge

1. Stand straight with your feet close together.

2. Step forward with the right foot, crossing it over the left leg. Your left heel comes off the ground and both legs form 90 degree angles. Keep your belly button pulled in and your chest up.

3. Step back to the starting position.

4. Next, step forward with your left foot, crossing it over your right leg. Right heel comes off the floor and your knees bend to 90 degrees.

5. Step back to the starting position. Continue alternating sides with each rep.

Burpee Jack

1. Start standing with your feet shoulder-width apart.

2. Squat down and place your hands on the ground directly under your shoulders.

3. Jump your feet back and together to get into a high plank with your back flat and body straight from head to heels. Abs are engaged.

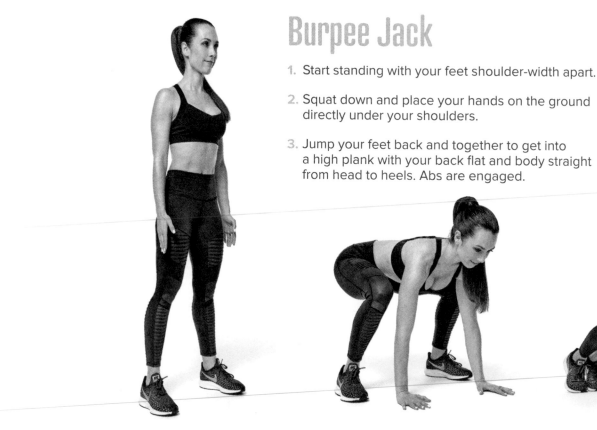

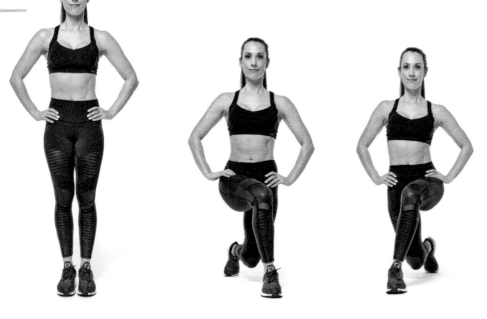

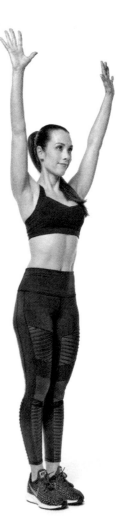

4. Next, jump your feet in, so they land outside of your hands. Make sure your heels are flat on the ground.

5. Jump up to a jumping jack, bringing feet together and arms above your head.

6. Jump your feet open to shoulder width and place your hands on the ground under your shoulders to begin your next rep.

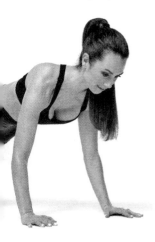

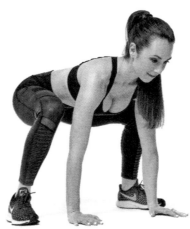

Cross-Country Skier to Ex Jump

1. Standing with feet together, jump and split your legs—right foot back, left foot forward—while raising your arms straight above your head.

2. Jump and split the legs again—left foot back, right foot forward—while bending your elbows to bring your arms down in front of you.

3. Next, ex jump by jumping and turning your body 90 degrees to the right with legs hip-width apart and jumping again, turning 180 degrees to the left.

4. Return to center and continue performing the sequence (cross-country skier to ex jump) for the duration of the set.

Two Side Shuffles to One Half-Skater

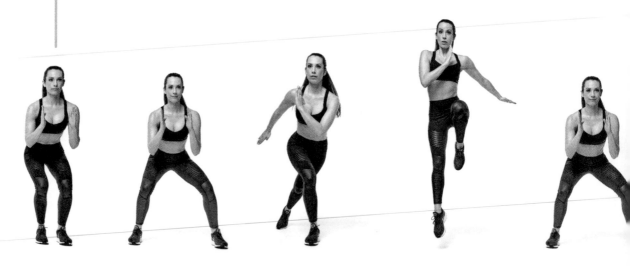

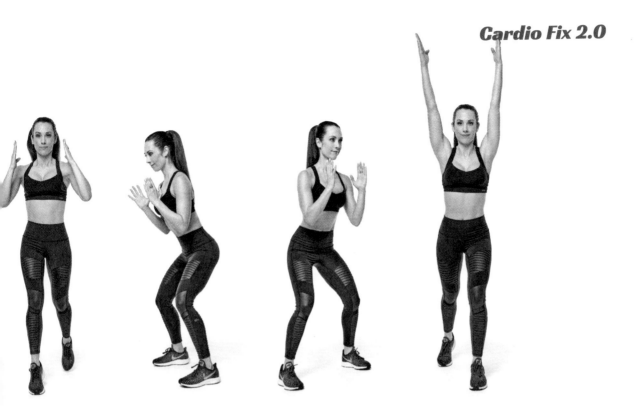

1. Start with feet hip-width apart and a slight bend in the knees, abs engaged, and chest lifted.

2. Take 2 shuffles to the right, and then swing both arms right as you cross your left leg behind you and tap the floor with your toes.

3. Drive your left knee up in front of you, hopping on your right leg.

4. Land softly and tap your left toes behind you again before shuffling two steps to your left.

5. Swing your arms to your left as you cross your right leg behind you, tap the floor with your toes, and then drive your right knee up, hopping on your left leg.

6. Land softly and tap the floor behind you again with your right toes. Continue moving back and forth for the duration of the set.

BONUS MOVE: Knee Pull, Up/Down, Hip Drop

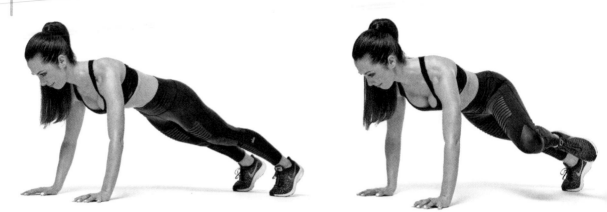

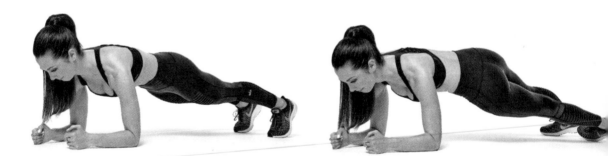

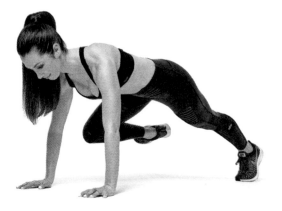

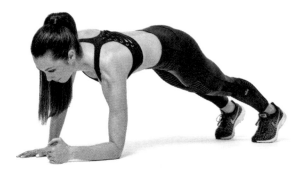

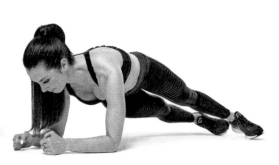

1. Start in a high plank: Hands on the floor under your shoulders, arms straight, feet hip-width apart, abs pulled in, and body straight.

2. Bend your left knee, bring it to your left elbow, and then return to the starting position. Repeat with your right leg.

3. Now, lower your left elbow to the ground so your forearm lies flat, then lower your right elbow to the ground.

4. From this elbow plank position, lower your left hip toward the ground by twisting your lower body and pivoting on your toes. Return to the elbow plank and then lower your right hip toward the ground.

5. Return to the high plank, pushing up first with your right arm and then left.

6. Repeat the sequence, this time starting with your right side. Continue alternating sides with each rep.

Warm-Up (3 minutes)

(Don't Skip This!)

Perform each warm-up move for 15 seconds. After completing the 6 moves, without resting, do a second round at a faster pace.

- **High Knees:** March in place, raising your knees as high as you can.

- **Jog in Place:** Bring your heels up toward your booty.

- **Jumping Jacks:** Do standard jumping jacks, just like in grade school.

- **Windmills:** With abs in and chest up, make wide circles with your straight arms. Halfway through, reverse the circle.

- **Over-the-Top Side Stretch:** With feet shoulder-width apart, raise your right arm toward the ceiling and do a side bend to the left. Reverse with the left arm to the right.

- **Alternating Toe Touch:** With feet shoulder-width apart, form a T with your torso by holding your arms out to your sides, parallel with the floor. Now swing your right arm down and bend at the waist to touch your right hand to your left toes. Return to start and repeat with your left hand to right toes.

Strength Exercises

Perform each move in pairs (or "supersets"), doing each move for 60 seconds and resting 30 seconds between them. Do each superset twice. Finish with the cooldown.

1. Squat to Rotating Shoulder Press
2. Hinge Row Curl

3. Sumo Overhead Triceps Extension
4. Push-up to Knee Tuck

5. Alternating Front Lunge with Front Deltoid Raise
6. Reverse Lunge with Lateral Deltoid Raise

7. Side Plank with Hip Drop and Leg Raise
8. Marching Crunch

Cooldown (3 minutes)
- Slow jog
- High knees
- Windmills (arm circles)
- Step side to side and shake out the arms.

Squat to Rotating Shoulder Press

1. Stand with feet shoulder-width apart holding a light dumbbell in each hand, racked at your shoulders.

2. Sit your butt back to squat until your thighs are parallel with the ground. Press your feet into the floor to straighten your legs.

3. As you drive up, press the left dumbbell above your head as you twist your torso to the right and pivot on your left toes. Keep your abs engaged.

4. Return to center into a squat, and then drive up, pressing the dumbbell in your right hand overhead while twisting left and pivoting on your right toes.

5. Return to a squat and repeat, alternating left and right.

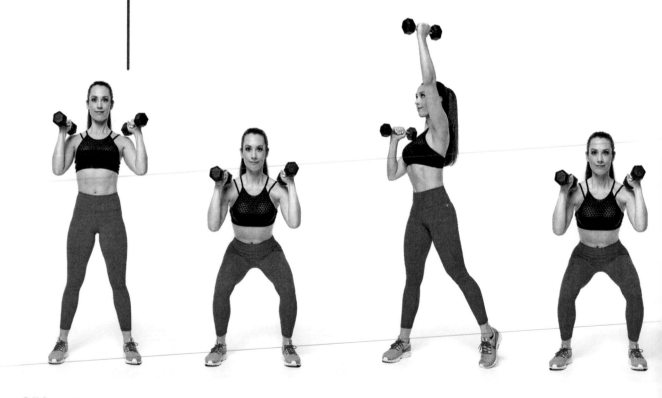

Note: Maintain a firm grip of the weights for safety.

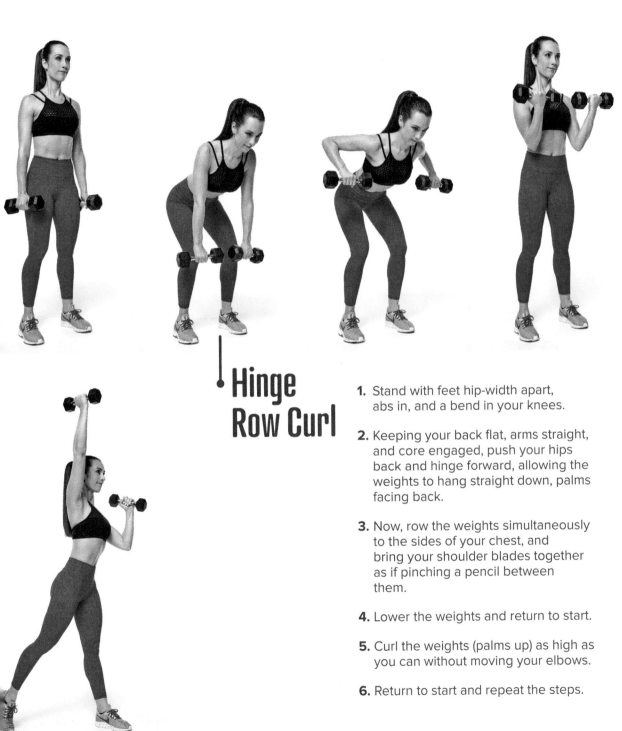

Hinge Row Curl

1. Stand with feet hip-width apart, abs in, and a bend in your knees.

2. Keeping your back flat, arms straight, and core engaged, push your hips back and hinge forward, allowing the weights to hang straight down, palms facing back.

3. Now, row the weights simultaneously to the sides of your chest, and bring your shoulder blades together as if pinching a pencil between them.

4. Lower the weights and return to start.

5. Curl the weights (palms up) as high as you can without moving your elbows.

6. Return to start and repeat the steps.

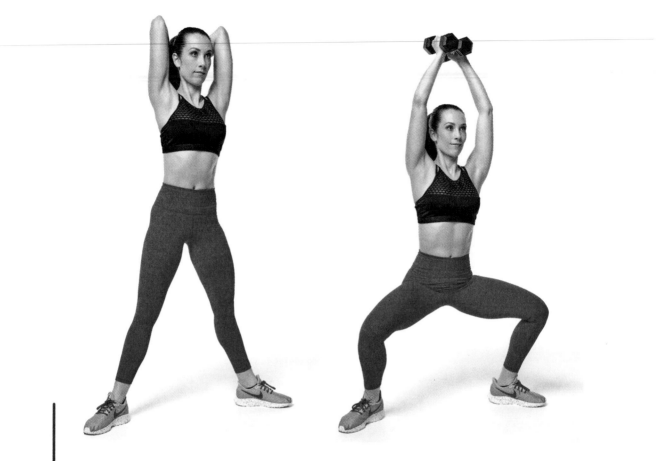

Sumo Overhead Triceps Extension

Note: Maintain a firm grip of the weights for safety.

1. Stand with feet set wider than shoulder-width apart and toes pointed outward. Raise both dumbbells above and behind your head, elbows bent 90 degrees.

2. As you bend your legs into a squat, extend your arms straight to raise the weights over your head, squeezing your elbows toward your ears. Your knees should track over your big toe. Don't allow them to collapse in.

3. Return to the starting position, straightening your legs and squeezing your inner thighs as you bend your elbows to lower the weights behind your head. Do this slowly, with control. Repeat.

Push-up to Knee Tuck

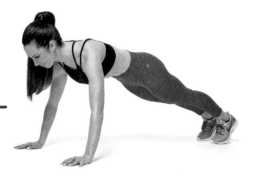

1. Assume a push-up position with your hands just outside your shoulders, feet together, abs in, and body straight.

2. Bend your elbows to lower your body toward the ground. When your chest touches the floor, straighten your arms.

3. Bring your left knee and then your right knee toward your chest. Perform another push-up.

4. Continue repeating the entire sequence.

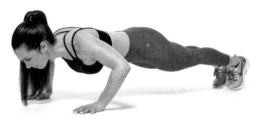

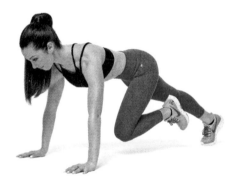

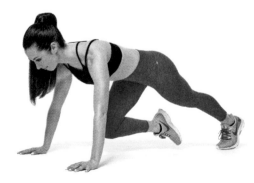

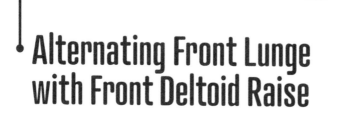

Alternating Front Lunge with Front Deltoid Raise

1. Stand with feet together, dumbbells held at your sides, palms facing in.

2. Keeping your core engaged and arms straight, step forward with your right leg, raising the dumbbell in your left hand to shoulder height in front of you as you lower your body until both knees are bent about 90 degrees (don't let your rear knee touch ground).

3. Reverse the movement to the starting position, and repeat, this time stepping forward with your left leg and raising the right dumbbell in front of you.

4. Continue alternating sides.

Reverse Lunge with Lateral Deltoid Raise

1. Stand with feet together, dumbbells held at your sides, palms facing in.

2. Step back into a reverse lunge with your right leg while raising the dumbbell held in your left hand out to your side to shoulder height. Your legs should be bent at 90-degree angles.

3. Lower the weight as you step back to the starting position.

4. Repeat, this time stepping back with your left leg and raising the dumbbell in your right hand.

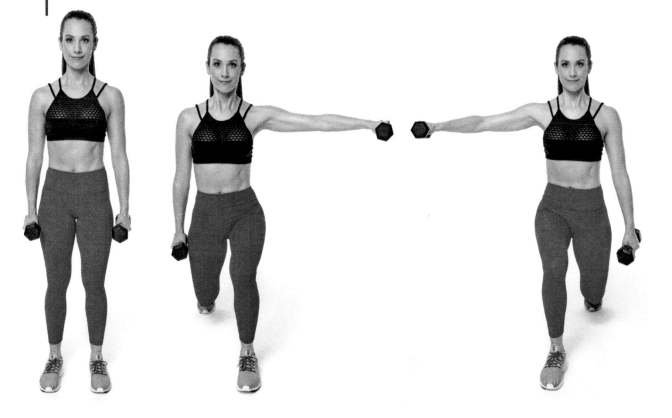

Side Plank with Hip Drop and Leg Raise

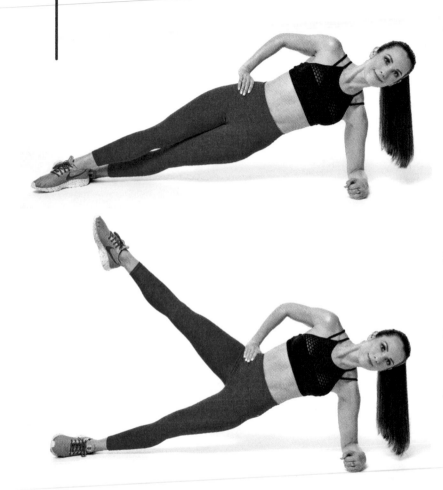

1. Lie on your left forearm and support your body with your left elbow directly under your left shoulder; your left forearm is flat on the floor, perpendicular to your body. Your feet should be staggered, not stacked. Raise your hips off the ground so that your body is straight.

2. Now, lift your right leg toward the ceiling. Hold for a second, then lower the leg.

3. Lower your hips to the floor, and then raise them again.

4. Repeat the entire sequence for 30 seconds, switch sides, and repeat.

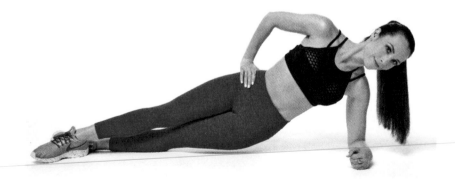

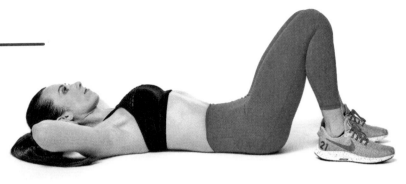

Marching Crunch

1. Lie flat on your back with knees bent and feet flat on the floor. Place your hands lightly behind your ears but not pulling on the neck. Tighten your abs and press your lower back down so there's no space between the floor and lower back.

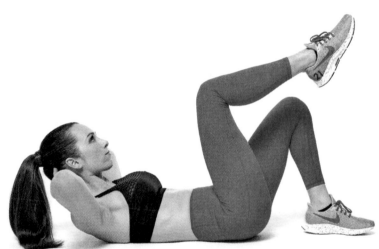

2. Each time you crunch, you march. Contract your abs to lift your head and shoulders off of the floor, simultaneously lifting one leg in a "marching" motion. Alternate legs with each rep.

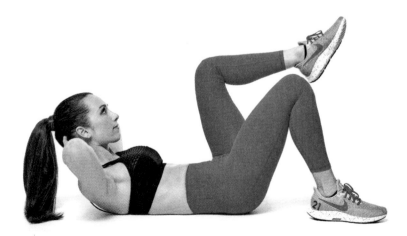

WHAT'S NEXT?

Congratulations on completing your first 30 days of *Lose Weight Like Crazy*. This isn't the end; it's just the beginning. Now that you know how the plan works, and you have the first month under your belt, it's time to dial it in even more. If you would like more information on how to do that, make sure you check out my *Ultimate Portion Fix* nutrition program on Beachbody On Demand. If you're ready to dial those workouts up, now is the perfect time to try *21 Day Fix* or *80 Day Obsession*.

So, what happens now? Below are your next steps, as well as some tips you can follow to be sure you continue making progress on this journey.

RECALCULATE: Every 30 days you need to recalculate your formula to make sure you stay in the proper bracket to continue losing weight. Your bracket can change from month to month, based on how much weight you lose, so don't forget to recalculate. The formulas start on page 130.

Once you've reached your ideal weight, you need to shift to maintenance. This will help you maintain your new healthy weight. To calculate your maintenance formula, first decide if you will be exercising and how much, or if you will continue this journey with minimal to no exercise. Your maintenance formulas are below.

Maintenance Formula for Moderate Exercise

(30 to 40 minutes per day at least 5 days a week of moderate to intense exercise)

Body Weight x 11 = Caloric Baseline

Caloric Baseline + 400 = Maintenance Calories

Maintenance Formula for Not Exercising

(or exercising 4 days a week or less for 30 minutes or less)

Body Weight x 11 = Caloric Baseline / Maintenance Calories

How do you know if you are at your ideal weight?

This can be tricky. I see so many people pick a random number and decide that when they weigh that number they will be at their ideal weight, or they will feel good about their body. Often, when I ask people where they came up with this number, they will say something like, "That's what I weighed in high school" or, "That's what I weighed when I was a college athlete." Unless you are just out of high school, or you are still working out like you did as a college athlete, that is not a great way to determine what a healthy weight is for yourself. In high school your body is still growing and changing. Ladies, we are just coming into our childbearing years.

Your body does change over time, it will carry weight differently, especially if you've already had one or more children. This doesn't mean you can't have an incredible figure; it just means we need to be careful about the number we are aiming for on the scale. A better way to determine an ideal weight is to find your healthy body fat percentage.

- **For woman,** a body fat percentage between 21% and 24% is considered fit, although athletes tend to skew lower (14% to 20%). Anything below 14% body fat is considered underweight for women.

- **For men,** the "fit" range is a bit lower (14% to 17% body fat) with athletes typically having between 6% and 13%. Anything below 6% is considered underweight for men.

These are all average recommendations. Everyone is built differently and will carry weight differently. It's best to check with your doctor to get a better idea of what is right for you.

You can have your body fat percentage checked in a few different ways. You can get a DEXA scan. DEXA (dual-energy x-ray absorptiometry) is a means of measuring bone mineral density using spectral imagining.

There is also hydrostatic body fat testing, sometimes referred to as a dunk tank. You are placed underwater for 5 seconds and your body fat percentage is measured. Because you are submerged, it doesn't mistake water weight for fat, like a lot of other tests do.

There are a lot of scales that can measure body fat as well. They're not as accurate as the methods mentioned above, but they can give you a decent idea of the range that you are in.

What To Do If You're Not Making Progress

First of all, take a deep breath; we're in this together. I've been with you from the beginning of this journey, and I'm not going to leave you stranded now. You might feel like you're not losing weight, or you're not losing weight fast enough, or you've hit a plateau. Here's what you need to know and what you can do to keep progressing.

If you feel like you are not losing weight fast enough, or you haven't lost weight in a few weeks and you're not sure why, here is what could be going on. Your body will ebb and flow with its weight loss. If you lost several pounds in the first week or two of starting the program, your body might slow the weight-loss process down for a week or two to make sure it's not in any kind of serious danger. Think about it: If you lose 5 pounds in the first week of this program, and then another 2 or 3 pounds in the second week, that's 8 pounds in a short period of time. Depending on your size, if your body continued to lose weight at that rate every week, it could be in trouble rather quickly. Our bodies are very smart. They will do what they need to protect us and make sure nothing is seriously wrong. So, if you lose a lot of weight in the first week or 2, it's normal for the body to slow down and only lose a pound or 2 (or maybe not lose anything) for the next week or 2 while it makes sure that everything is OK. Once your body realizes it's not starving, or continuing to drop large amounts of weight at a rapid pace, the weight loss will usually kick back in. So, be patient.

Other things to look at if you feel you aren't losing weight or aren't losing weight fast enough:

Are you using the proper formula?

You may have gone into the program with the best of intentions, planning on exercising 5 days a week for an hour a day, so you used the formula for extremely challenging exercise. But, after the first few days, you realized your schedule is very busy and all you can make time for is 30 minutes a day, 5 days a week. Did you adjust the formula to that of moderate intensity exercise? This will impact your results, so make sure you use the proper formula.

My next question is: Are you trying to outsmart the science of the program? I see it all the time. Someone calculates their formula for weight loss and they find they are in plan C. They decide that to lose weight even faster they will just drop down to plan B. Eat less, lose more, right? WRONG! By dropping down to a lower bracket, you put yourself at too big of a deficit. Now your body is fighting for the calories and nutrients it needs to perform daily activities, so instead of losing weight, it holds on to everything it's given to make sure it has enough energy. Don't switch brackets just because you think it will help you lose weight faster. Don't cut out containers because you think carbs are bad or make you hold on to weight. Trust the process and the program. It works if you do the work.

Other things to look at:

- **Continue to use your containers for measuring your food.** As you lose weight, it's important not to get complacent with the tools you've been given.

- **Continue tracking your containers.** Pay attention to where on the food list your food choices are coming from. It should be coming from the top one-third of the food lists 85% to 90% of the time.

- **Don't overdo treat substitutions.** No more than 3 times per week.

- **Eat your containers and only your containers.** It's important to take an honest look at what you're eating during the week. Have you been eating off of your kids' plates? Did you go out with friends for happy hour and eat chips while sipping a cocktail but not account for them? Did you have a few extra bites while cooking dinner? It all adds up.

- **Drink half of your body weight in ounces of water each day.**

- **Get plenty of sleep.**

- **Practice self-care.**

Congratulations! You now have the tools you need to lose weight like crazy no matter what this crazy life throws at you, and it will throw things at you. It will test you and push you outside of your comfort zone. Don't fear the challenges, embrace them. They are there to help you grow into the best possible version of yourself. Remember, there are no failures, only redirects. Your path directed you to this book, to this plan. You can have amazing success with it, if you put in the work. There is no end date on living a healthy life. It's not just for 30 days or 60 days; it's a journey that spans a lifetime. There will be good days and hard days. I will end this by once again encouraging you to focus on progress, not perfection; it will make the journey a whole lot more enjoyable.

Away we go!

Acknowledgments

I'd like to thank Beachbody CEO Carl Daikeler for taking a chance on me when no one else would. Thank you for allowing me the opportunity to live my dream of helping others live healthier lives. You have given me a platform on which to learn, grow, and create. I am forever grateful for the opportunities, the lessons, your mentorship, and your friendship. I can't wait for what's next with my Beachbody family.

I'd like to thank my brother Bobby Calabrese for not only creating the 23 delicious recipes in this book but for all the fantastic recipes you have created and continue to create. You truly are an evil genius; I don't know how you do it but I'm so happy that you do. Thank you for being my co-host on our cooking show *FIXATE*, making me laugh on long days, and lifting me up on hard days. Thank you for also helping me write this book. It would not be what it is without you.

Thank you to my dad, Robert Calabrese, for raising me to be a strong, independent woman who knows what she wants and goes after it with everything she has. Thank you for teaching me that I could do anything I set my mind to. Thank you for all the love and the lessons; watching you do hard things taught me that I could do them, too.

Thank you to my family: my mom, Mary, sister Calie, brother Jon, sister Kat, my aunts, my uncles, cousins, and grandparents for always being there for me and going on this crazy journey we call life together. I love each and every one of you.

Thank you to my Beachbody family; you are my home away from home, and my second family. I could not do all that I have done without the enormous team of support I have behind me every day. Their names aren't in the spotlight, their faces aren't on the cover of my workout programs or books, but without them I couldn't do it.

Last but definitely not least, thank you to my fans, my followers, the millions of people who have trusted me to take them on a journey to better health. I'm thanked all the time by people for changing their lives, but really you all have changed mine. You inspire me daily to keep pushing, keep creating, to never give up. I've given you the tools but YOU did the work. I will always work to be the best version of me to hopefully inspire you to be the best version of you.

Index

Note: Page numbers in *italics* indicate recipes.